Beautiful!

Images of Health, Joy, and Vitality
in Pregnancy and Birth

By Jennie Joseph
Pregnancy and Family photos by Alejandra Sarmiento

Proceeds from the sale of this book will go towards continuing the clinical work of the center,
our midwifery and educational programs, and the sharing of The JJ Way® maternal child health system across the USA.

Beautiful!

Images of Health, Joy, and Vitality
in Pregnancy and Birth

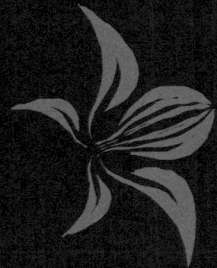

I dedicate this book to my family, with gratitude and love.

You too are beautiful – thank you.

My husband Ellison James Eady Jr.

My son Luke Eady

My parents Eric and Sylvia Joseph

My siblings Carol Collier, Frances Pack, and Eric Joseph Jr.

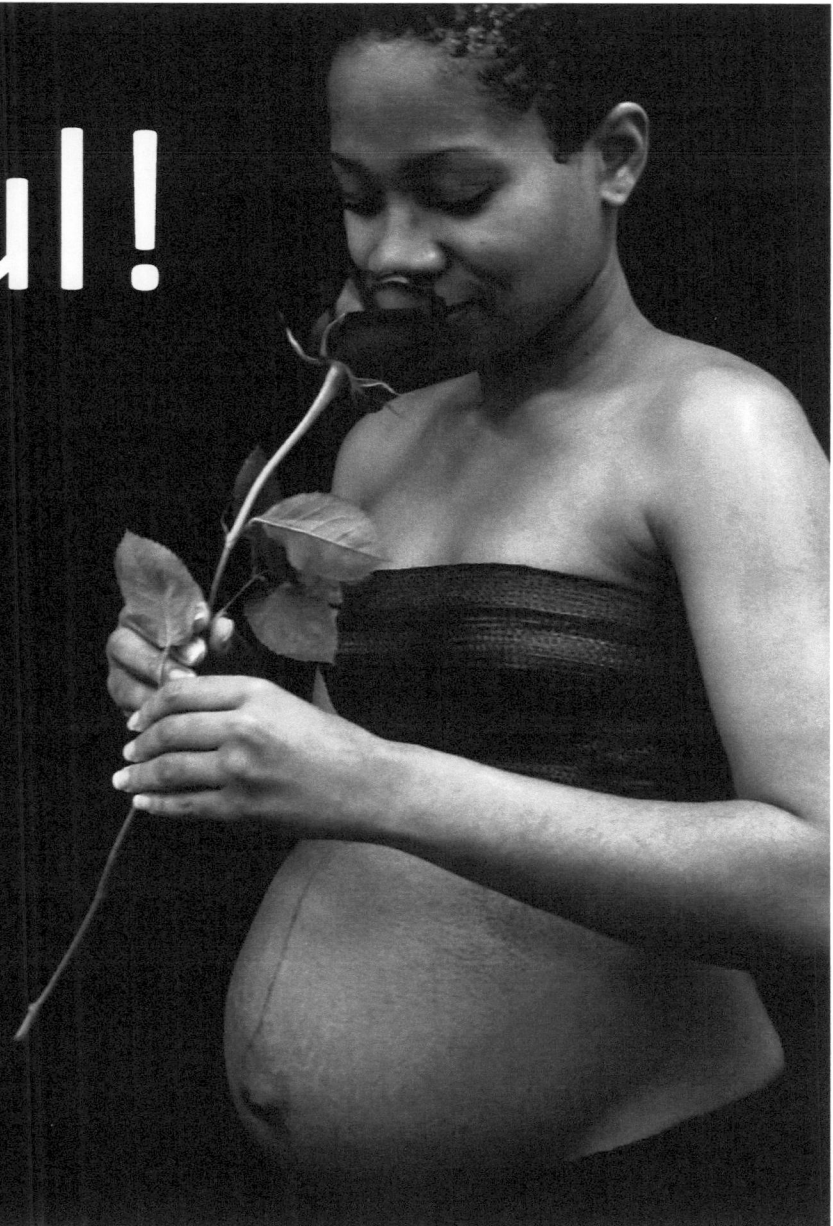

Beautiful! Images of Health, Joy, and Vitality in Pregnancy and Birth by Jennie Joseph

Published by Watersprings Publishing,
a division of Watersprings Media House, LLC.
P.O. Box 1284 Olive Branch, MS 38654
www.WaterspringsPublishing.com

Printed in the United States of America

ISBN-13: 979-8-9859594-3-7 (Hardcover)

Acknowledgments

Where do I begin? My late husband **James** whose steadfast support and unwavering belief carried me through the early years, whose financial provision allowed countless families to receive unfunded care and whose ability to "let me be me" provided the foundation for the work I'm able to do today. Truly a midwife's husband. I love you and I miss you.

My son **Luke**, my only child, who sacrificed and shared me with so many other women and their children; who followed me from home to home, center to center, office to office, waiting patiently as demand for my practice grew and took me further away from my own family. I love you too, and I thank you.

To the multitude of women and babies who have touched my life, to every single one of you. I say thank you to those of you whose images grace this book. I acknowledge you for your beauty and thank you for your heart. To every patient that has come through our doors or has been touched by The JJ Way® in action, I appreciate your trust and belief in my system - thank you.

Deep gratitude to **Alejandra Sarmiento** whose amazing photography inspired me to create this book. Her talent and artistry led me to believe that I could tell The JJ Way® story without words - thank you.

To **Katrina Nelson, Dr. Chandra Adams** and The Birth Place clinical staff and students - both past and present, who faithfully followed every twist and turn with me, who stepped outside the box, who applied themselves and reinvented women's healthcare as The JJ Way® developed. Special thanks to Sally Ali, Kathy Bradley, Beth Lewis from the early days! The multitude of midwives and advocates, including Justine Clegg and Char Lynn, who along with Florida Governor Lawton Chiles initially opened the door to my receiving a Florida license as a foreign trained midwife. Grand Midwife Gladys Milton (deceased), her daughter Maria Milton, Alice Pillay and all the

Grand midwives on whose shoulders I stand, - I salute you.

To my cherished group of **Elder Midwives**, girlfriends and sistah friends, who have allowed me into their lives and taught me so much. Friends and family who have not wavered in their belief or encouragement are too numerous to mention but you know who you are - I have not forgotten any one of you.

To all in public health, in clinical practice, and in caring and supportive roles who toil daily inside a system that has allowed this maternal health injustice to happen to our communities, to those of you who didn't need this book to realize the dire circumstances we find ourselves in, to everyone who is already fighting or who will now stand up, seen or unseen, compensated or uncompensated - a heartfelt THANK YOU!

Introduction

I stepped off a transatlantic flight in Miami Florida on a brilliant May day in 1989, gathered my three-year-old son, our baggage and my courage and strode purposefully out of the airport into the unfamiliar heat to begin my new life as a Florida resident and American wife. I left behind family, friends and familiarity but having found the man of my dreams I knew what I had to do. I was ready for my future and excited about the possibilities. My West Indian heritage intermingled with my British upbringing, not to mention my many previous international travels, had prepared me for anything America would throw at me. Even now, looking back on 32 years in America I now know that nothing could have really prepared me for what I was going to face.

I had been a midwife since 1981, trained in a busy maternity hospital in the London suburbs and accustomed to total acceptance of birth as a normal life event with low-risk women being attended by midwives for all aspects of their care. Totally unaware of the American health care system I fully expected to find a job in a local hospital or clinic, to pick up where I left off practicing the only profession I'd ever known or loved since the age of 19 - Midwifery. A few years later, frustrated, and disappointed that Midwifery was not mainstream, I turned to independent home birth as a way to continue my passion and I began a small practice serving Central Florida families. In that time, I learned a lot. I have always operated from the simple premise that every woman wants a healthy baby, and every woman deserves one. The opportunity for growth and development of all concerned, physically, emotionally, psychologically, and spiritually is phenomenal during the childbearing cycle. Women, families, and communities all benefit from the life altering events that surround bringing a healthy pregnancy to term. Sadly, that has not been my American Experience. There is a distinct difference in birth outcomes for women of color in the United States. Simply put, between two to three times as many Black babies as compared to white are born too soon, too small, or will die before reaching their first birthday. Three to four times as many Black and Indigenous women die due to childbirth related complications, while tens of thousands nearly die or are harmed due to preventable causes in the US today. There are even worse statistics in certain urban or rural pockets throughout the country, but overall, nationally the racial disparities stand. Infant mortality is a measure of how well a country is faring in the realm of health and such discouraging figures and egregious birth outcomes have the United States ranking last among all other industrial nations.

What could be behind these awful statistics? Theories abound as to why prematurity, low birth weight, morbidity (poor health) and mortality have become a 'crisis' in the black community. Lack of access to healthcare, no insurance, low resources, little support, low socioeconomic status, social determinants of health and poor health prior to pregnancy have all been suggested. And yet the answers are simple and right in front of us - *racism, classism, sexism and discrimination are the root causes.* The research continues and the 'blame the mother' tropes abound leaving all concerned with a sense of powerless despair as year in and year out we grieve the preventable loss of our health, our babies, our promise, and our lives.

25 years ago, I realized I was unable to stand by and accept the status quo, so I searched for a solution that could make a difference for the women of color in my area. I knew that the midwifery model of providing healthcare, a centuries old standard of woman-to-woman care, can make an impact. Slowly I developed a program, a method, a system: The JJ Way® was born. I wanted practical, workable, affordable solutions to remove and reduce the obstacles to care. Simple, understandable, step-by-step directions, instructions and plans became the backbone of my program. Women and families were empowered, engaged, and supported as team members in the awesome task of reaching the goal of a full-term healthy baby. Lack of insurance or finances was not allowed to impact the quality, frequency, or availability of care. Word-of-

mouth spread and Commonsense Childbirth Inc., a non-profit organization was formed to meet the rapidly growing need. In credit to its success, here we are 25 years later still making an enormous difference today.

Commonsense Childbirth and The JJ Way® have continued to go from strength to strength. I have been able to set up a midwifery school, Commonsense Childbirth School of Midwifery, which is now the first private and nationally accredited Midwifery School owned and operated by a Black woman in the United States. In order to address the lack of access to safe, respectful, quality care experienced by marginalized communities I also established the Easy Access Clinic™ model for pregnant people who are most at risk of not receiving prenatal and postpartum care. There are several other clinics around the country on track to being accredited through our programs. Commonsense Childbirth Institute is training and diversifying the perinatal workforce on a national level - including doulas, childbirth educators, Lactation educators, and community health workers. Lastly, our movement building body, the National Perinatal Task Force, focuses on supporting and advocating for perinatal health and support service workers through collective care, collective leadership and workforce development via our national networks and community of practice.

I have been fortunate enough to have built up a voice, a loud voice, for families of color and have been able to speak to policy makers including the US Congress and Congressional briefings on Capitol Hill, health institutions, practitioners, and community stakeholders. I have traveled to raise awareness at Maternal Child Health conferences and given many media interviews on these important topics. I've been honored to serve in leadership positions amongst US and international Midwife movements and organizations. In 2022 I received the distinct honor of being named one of 12 women of the year for TIME Magazine. Despite all of this you will still find me helping people embrace The JJ Way®, whether patients or providers, while thoroughly enjoying the privilege of being part of *their* Incredible Journey to *their* full empowerment and joy.

Looking back, I can see how we got here. Our model has always made sure that pregnant people and their families were centered and that they knew that they were going to be supported no matter what. Utilizing the four JJ Way® tenets of **access, connections, knowledge,** and **empowerment** we set to work all those years ago. Our model has not changed, and our outcomes have proven over and over again that this model works. It takes meeting the mother where she is in her life without judging her or blaming her; empowerment and respect are key in all interactions. Listening attentively, open communication and easy access to staff without fear of criticism or humiliation can do wonders for overall health. Continuity of care with familiar providers encourages greater compliance with healthcare visits, follow-through with instructions and timely reporting of health concerns. Additionally, staff are empowered and encouraged to take ownership and leadership of their positions while they apply their own lived experience in empathetic, culturally safe ways, The JJ Way®

A particular JJ Way® component is the stated goal of a full-term baby, every person, every time. Thus, every woman, family member and friendly supporter is in no doubt as to the purpose of each prenatal visit. Every member of the newly formed team recognizes and acknowledges the woman as being fully competent to fulfill the role of motherhood and by encouraging prenatal bonding to the baby, all parties become entirely invested in the healthiest possible outcome. Coming together this way to provide wrap-around support helps pregnant people remain in their best all-round health, including mentally, emotionally, spiritually as well as physically. This naturally reduces the high morbidity and mortality rates and by doing so lessens the incidence of preventable high-risk situations developing or worsening, while markedly decreasing the overwhelming numbers of Black and Brown babies that need to go to the neonatal intensive care units if they survive. Mitigating these seemingly intractable conditions relieves the burden on the parents, families and communities and eliminates the long-term repercussions and runaway costs of this historical, structural and institutional injustice once and for all.

I developed this book in 2007 to showcase the beauty of the perinatal period. Each stage is wondrous and fascinating in its own way. I want pregnant women to be able to see a reflection of themselves, a comparison, and a similarity; for all of us to recognize and acknowledge the power, strength and endurance of women to bear children with dignity, even in desperate times, to remind ourselves that birth is not an illness and that a holistic, respectful approach to care is a morally feasible and cost-effective alternative that must be applied now. The women in these pictures are all from my practice, not models or professionals, simply women who fully embraced The JJ Way® in their own way and carried their babies to term. Black women from all walks of life with amazing and inspiring stories. Women that I was destined to meet along the way who showed me their courage, their willingness to stand for the health of their babies, the determination to change these horrendous statistics, and their mettle to face the odds head-on and win. Women who helped me grow personally and reminded me that if we move forward together we can do great things.

If you didn't know the egregious and worsening statistics that surround African American childbearing parents and their families in the USA, you do now. This book is a reminder for all of us that we **can** make a difference; that there **is** a way, a tangible way, an attainable way – the results of which are indeed Beautiful!

In this my 63rd year of life, and Commonsense Childbirth's 25th, I am encouraged. I present these images to you so the women can tell their own stories. See if you can see what I see...... the gift that is our legacy, our humanity, our promise. Commonsense Childbirth along with so many others in the USA today are building a movement to birth a more just and loving world. Join us!

— Jennie Joseph

1

Pregnancy

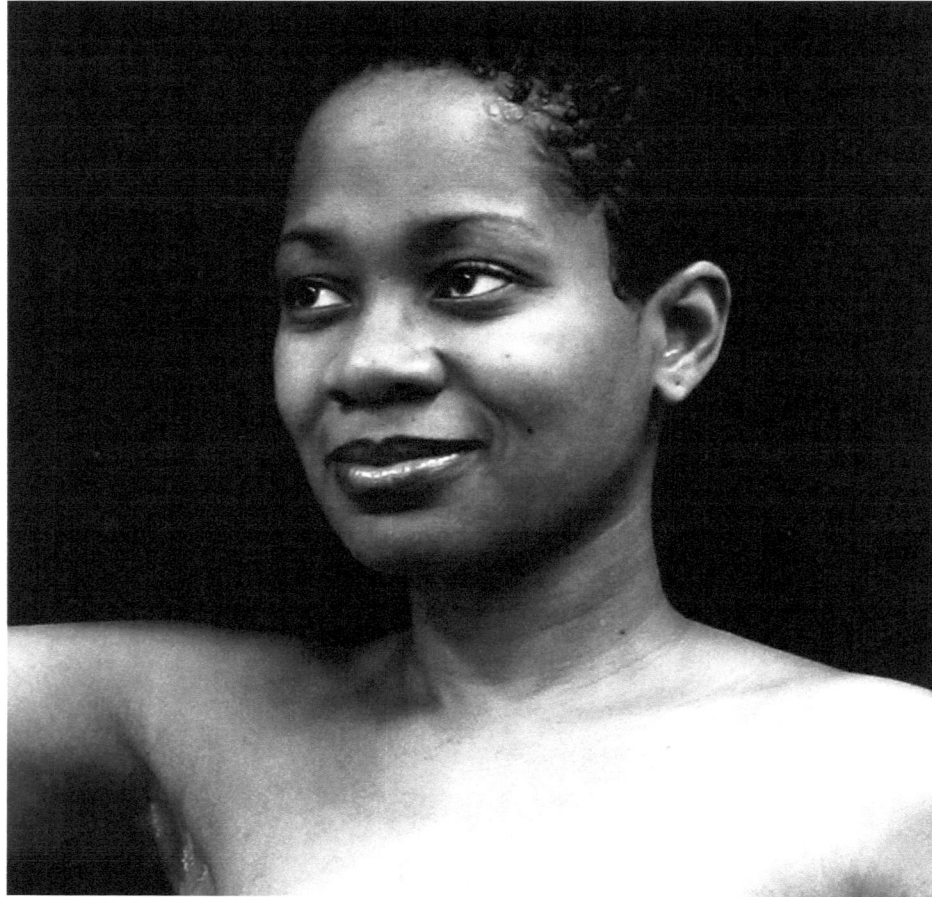

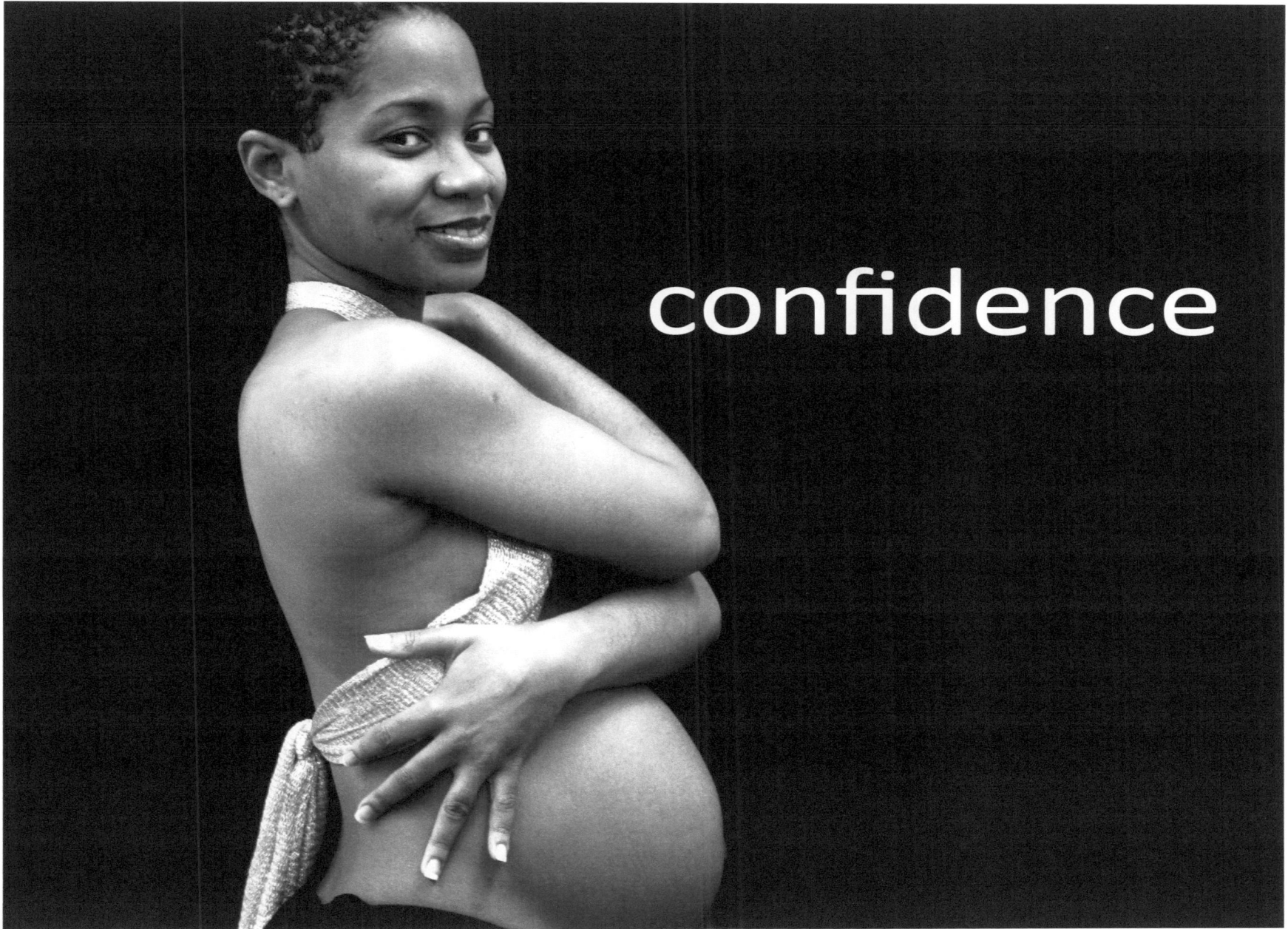

confidence

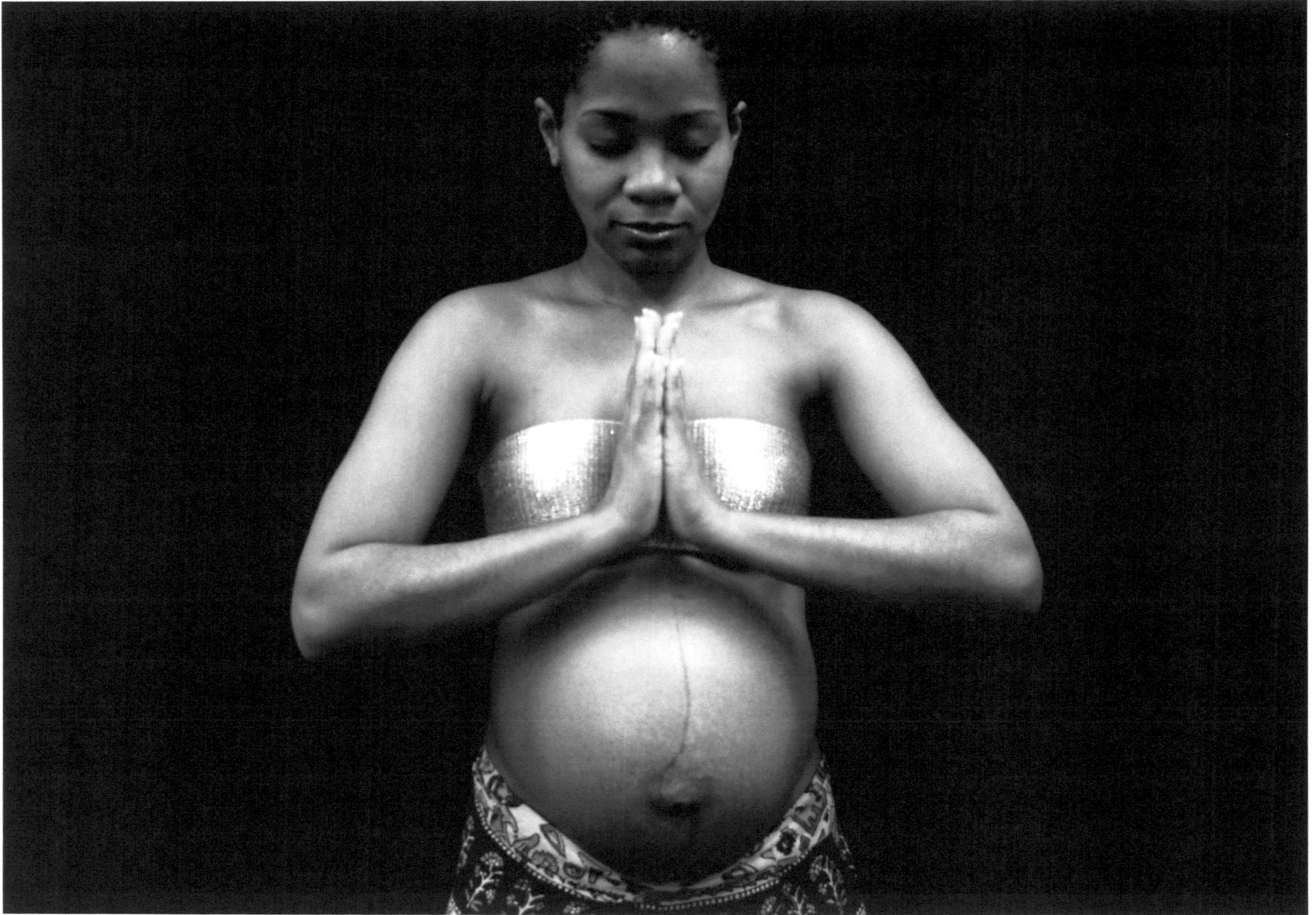

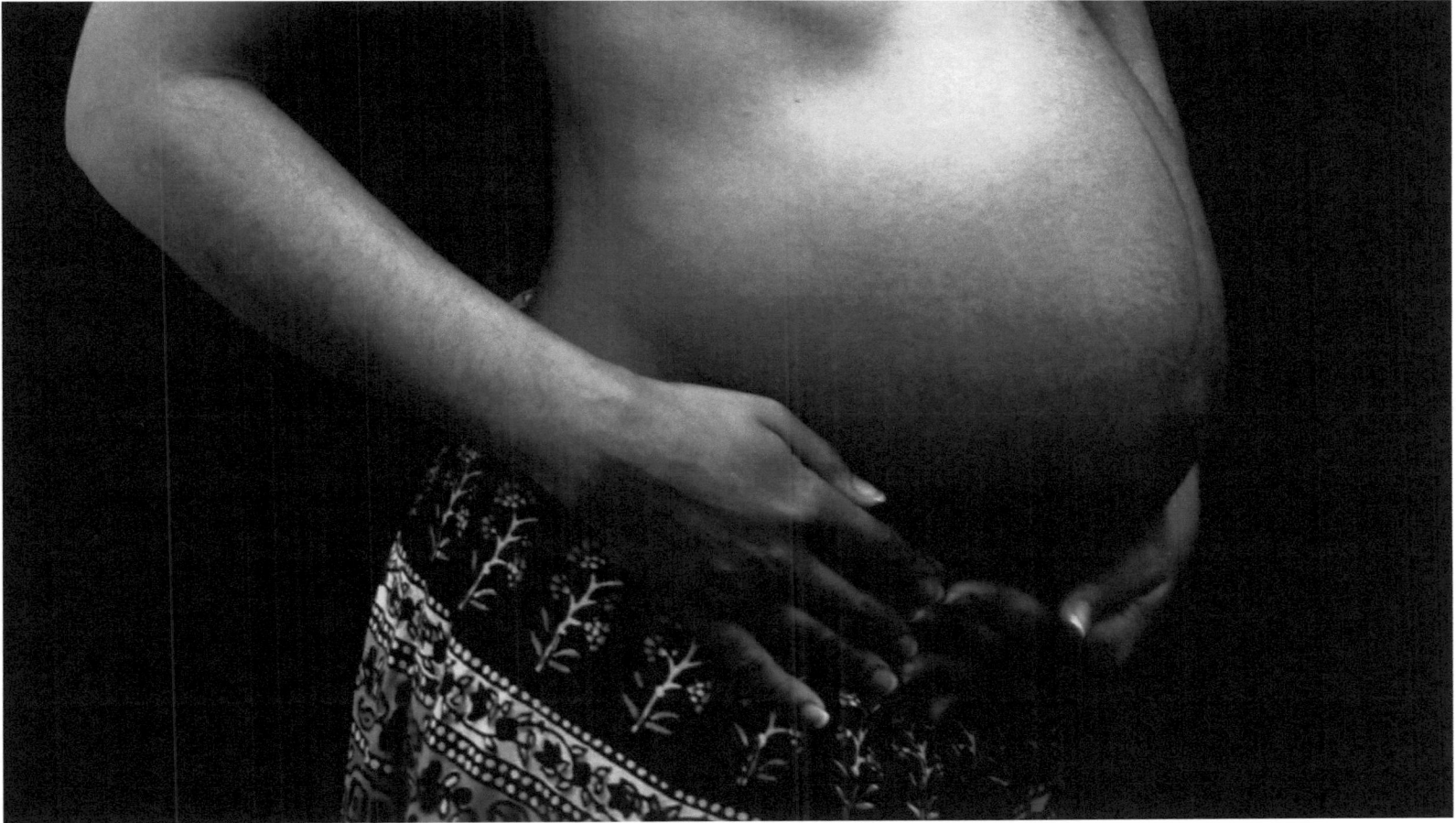

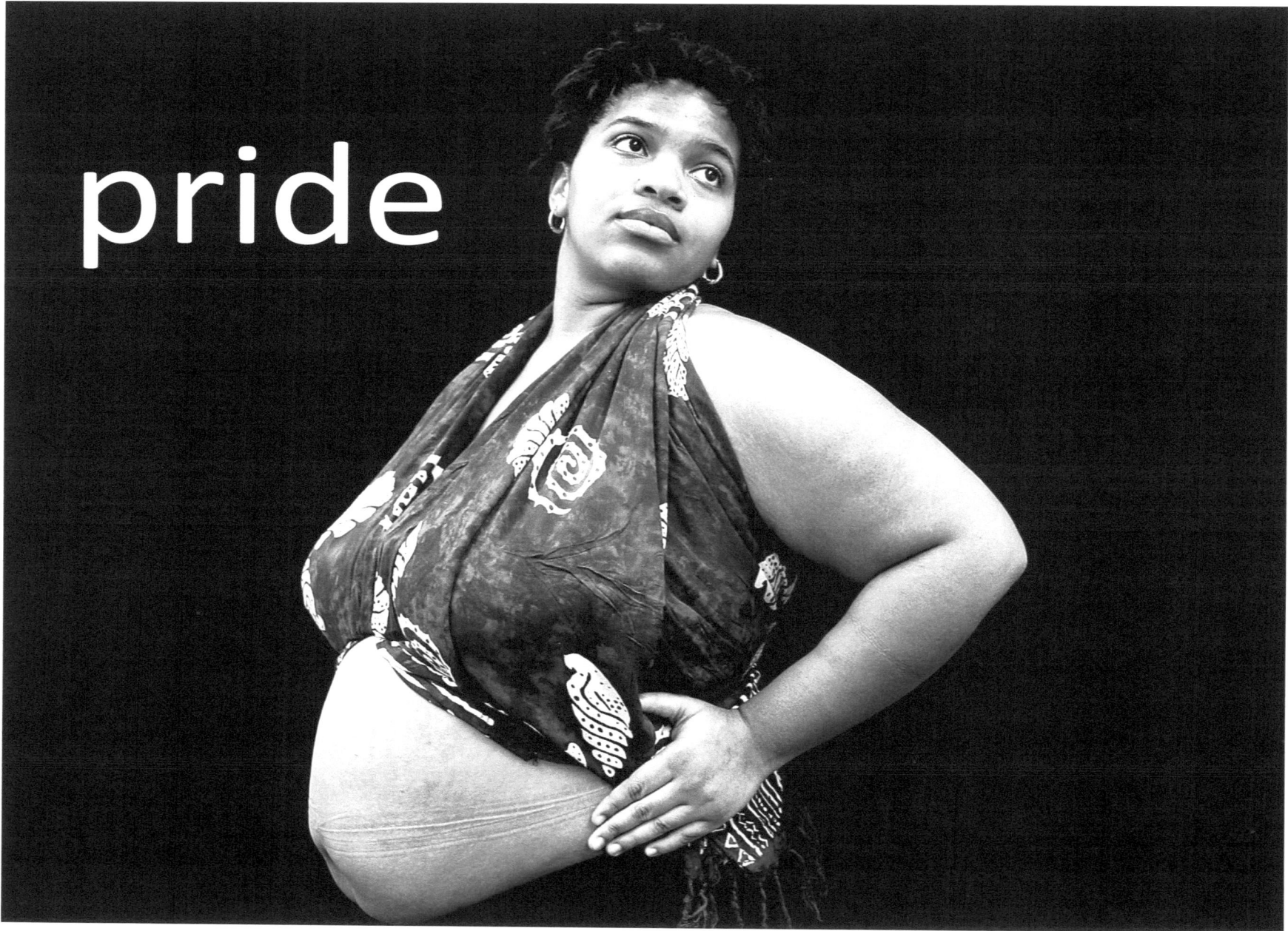

pride

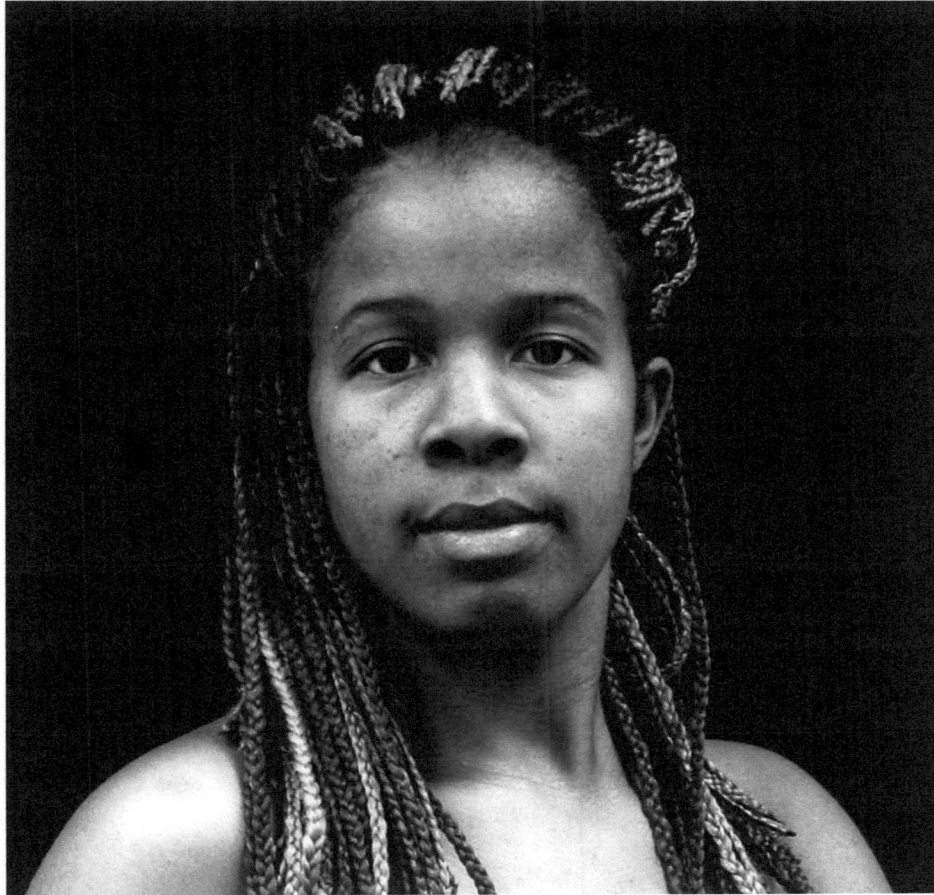

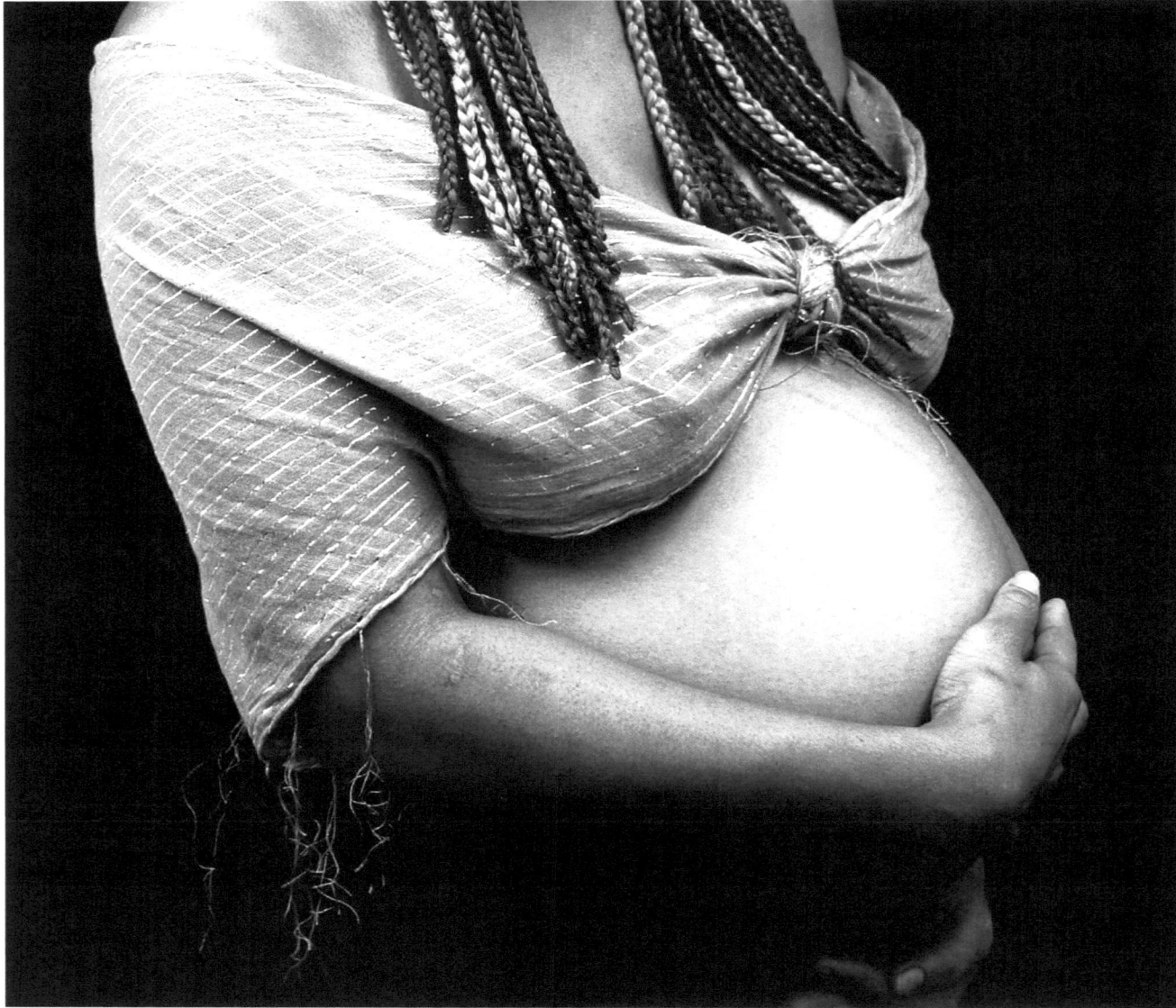

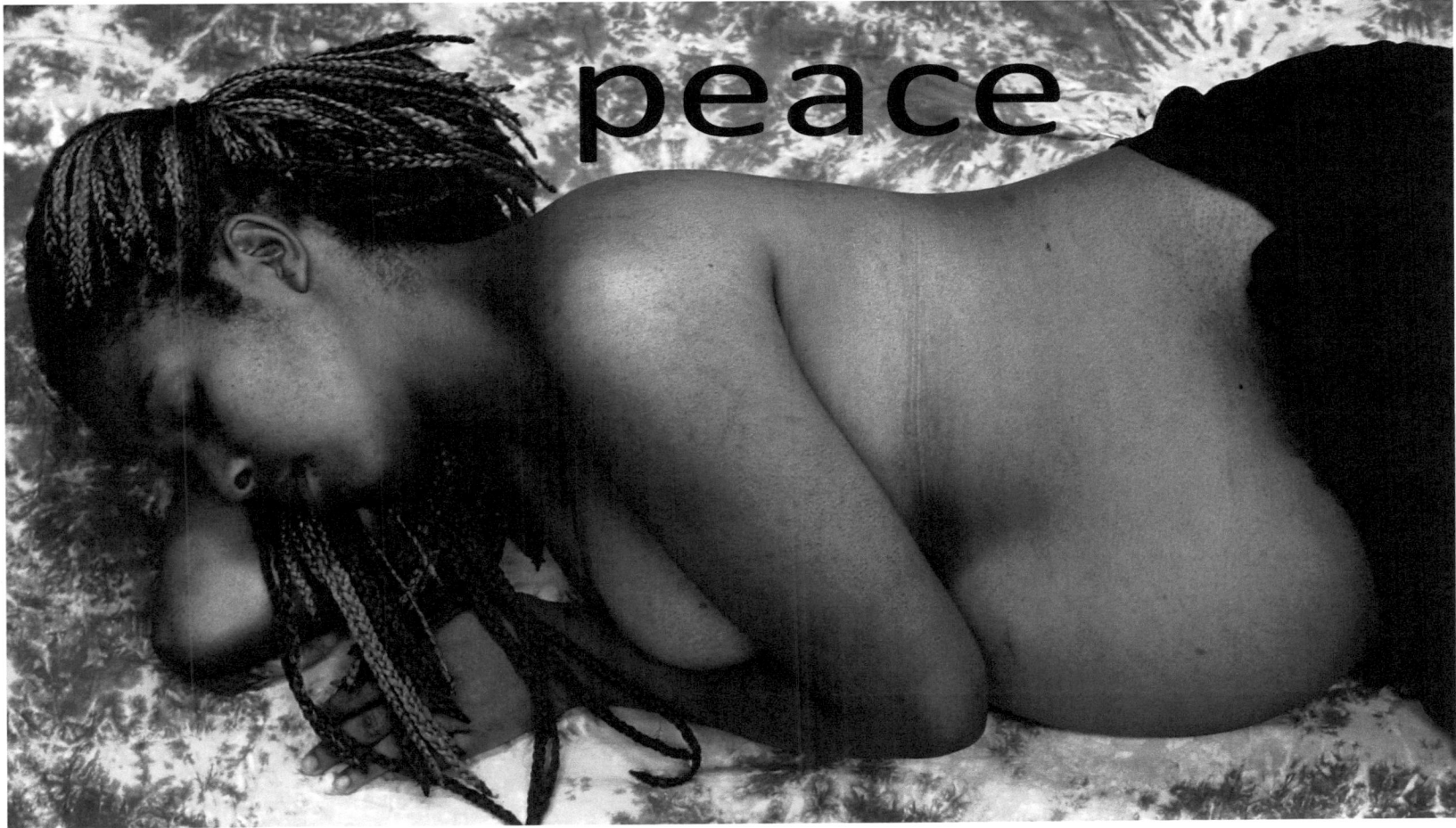

peace

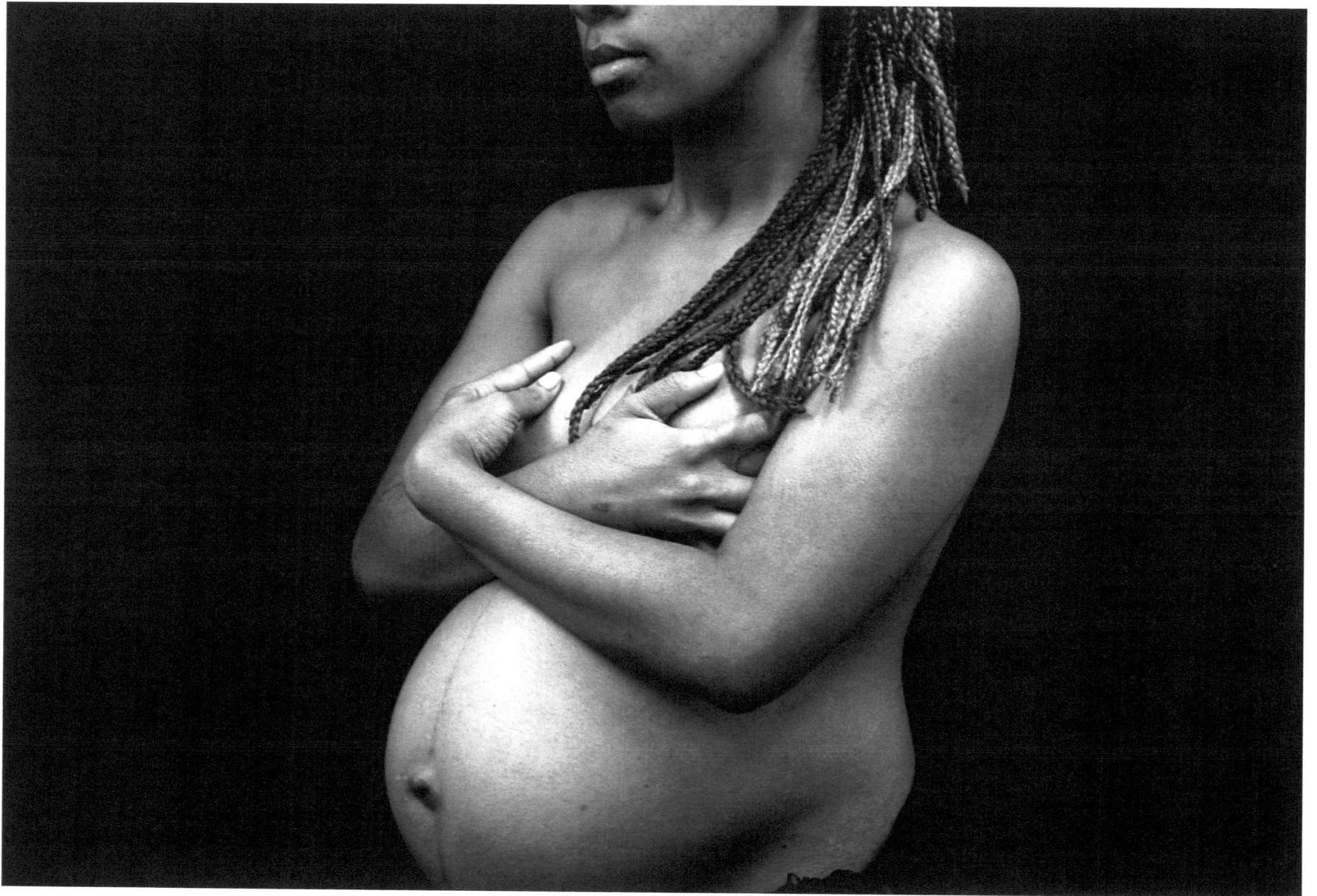

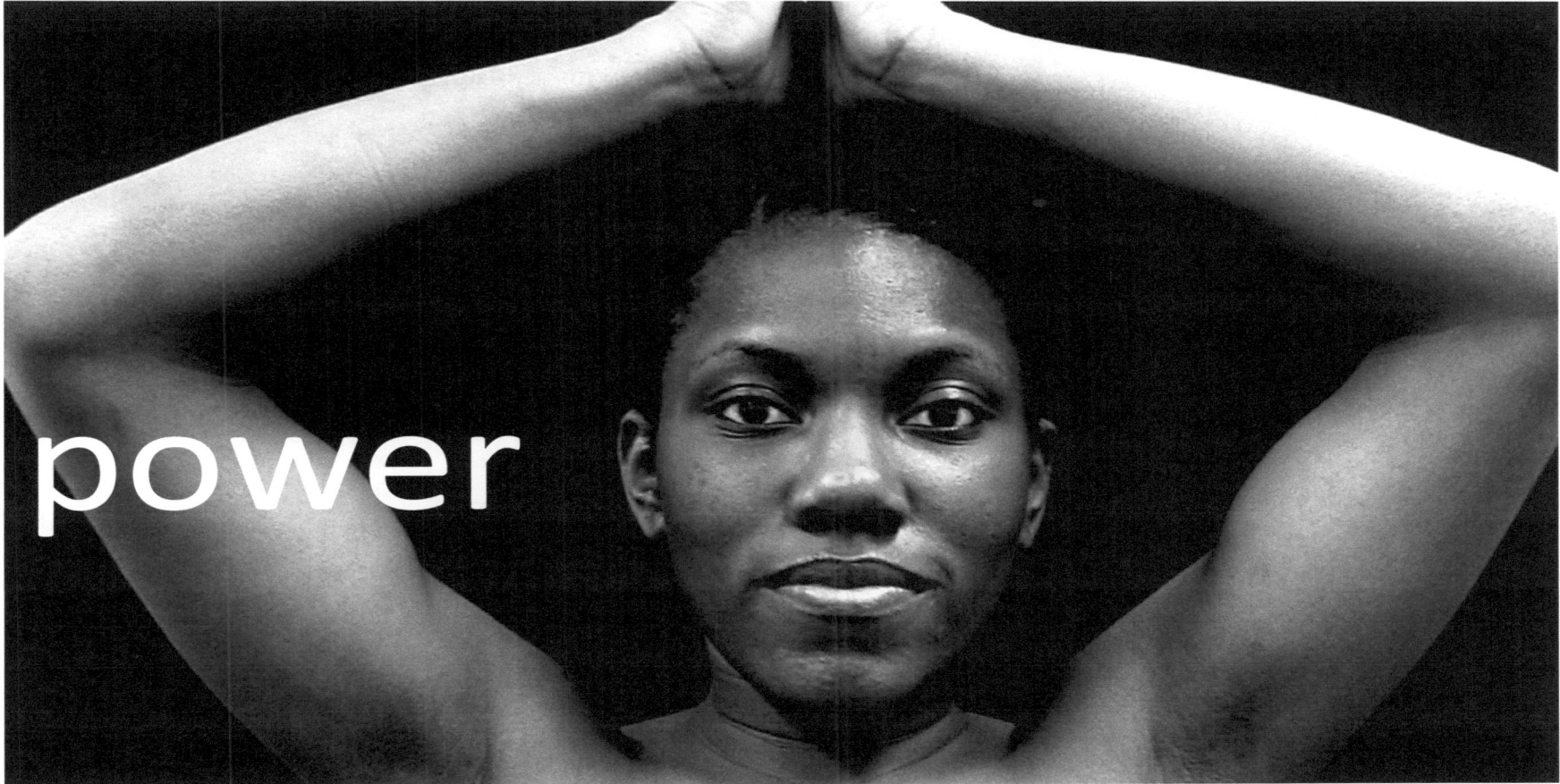

power

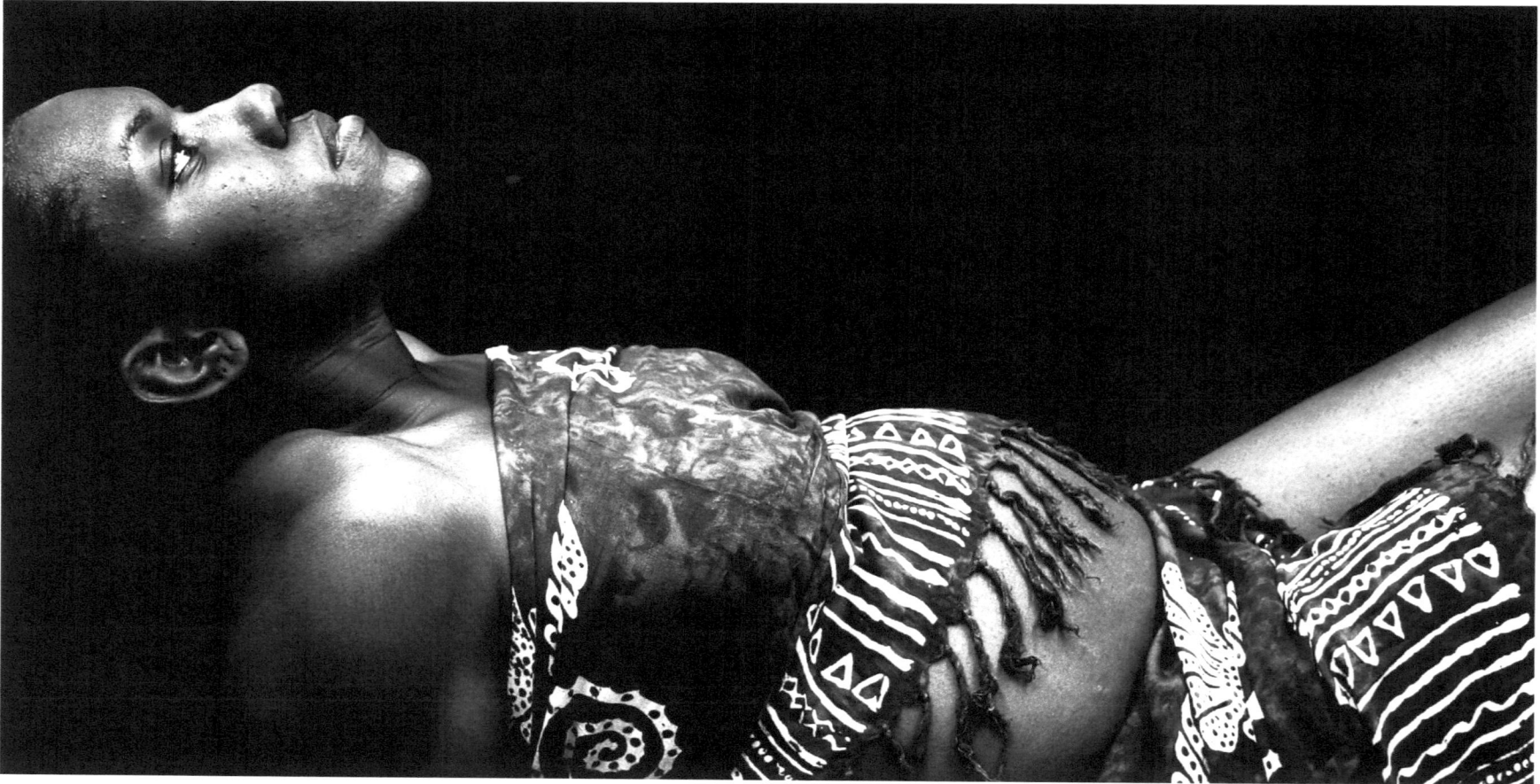

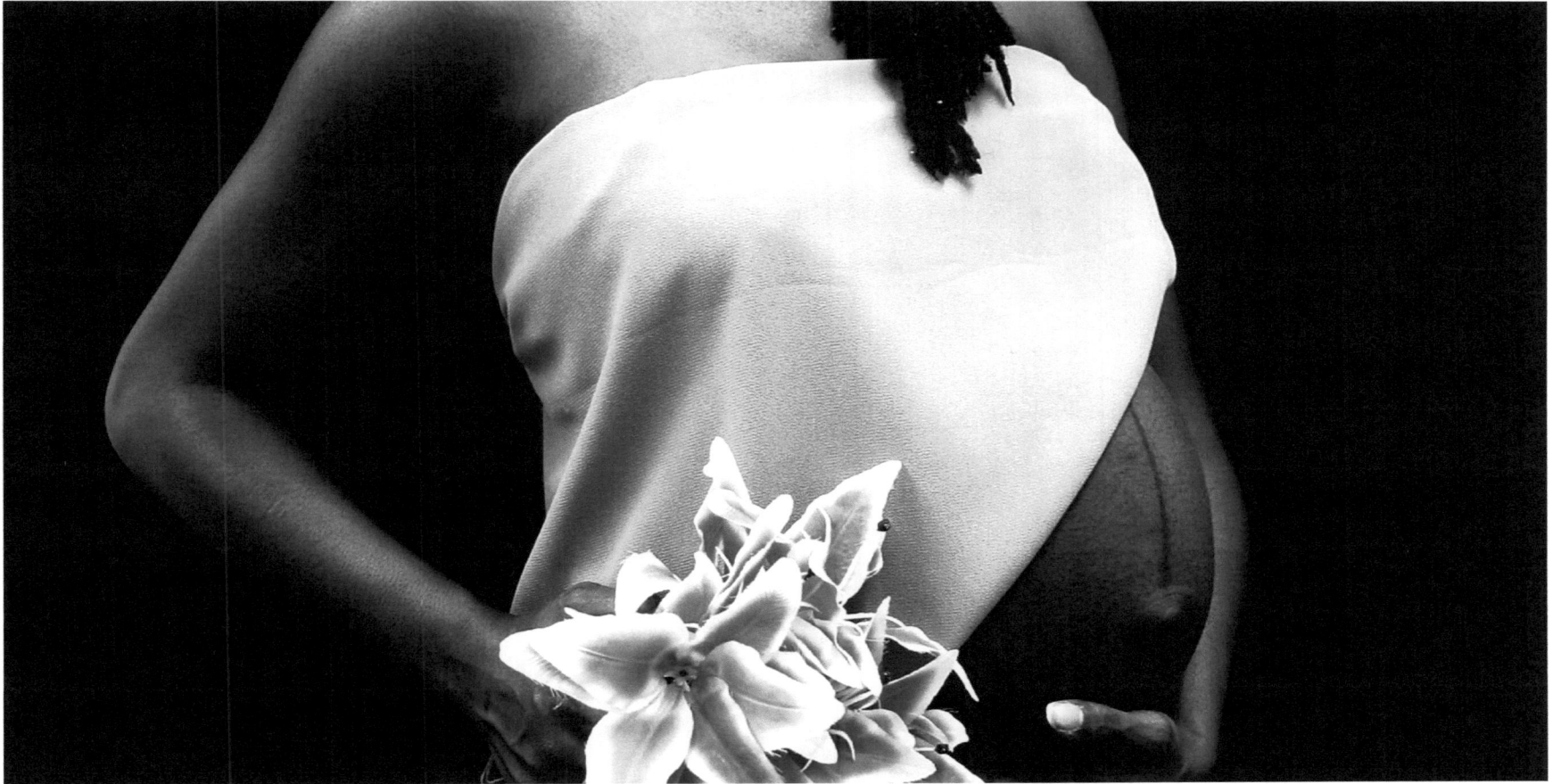

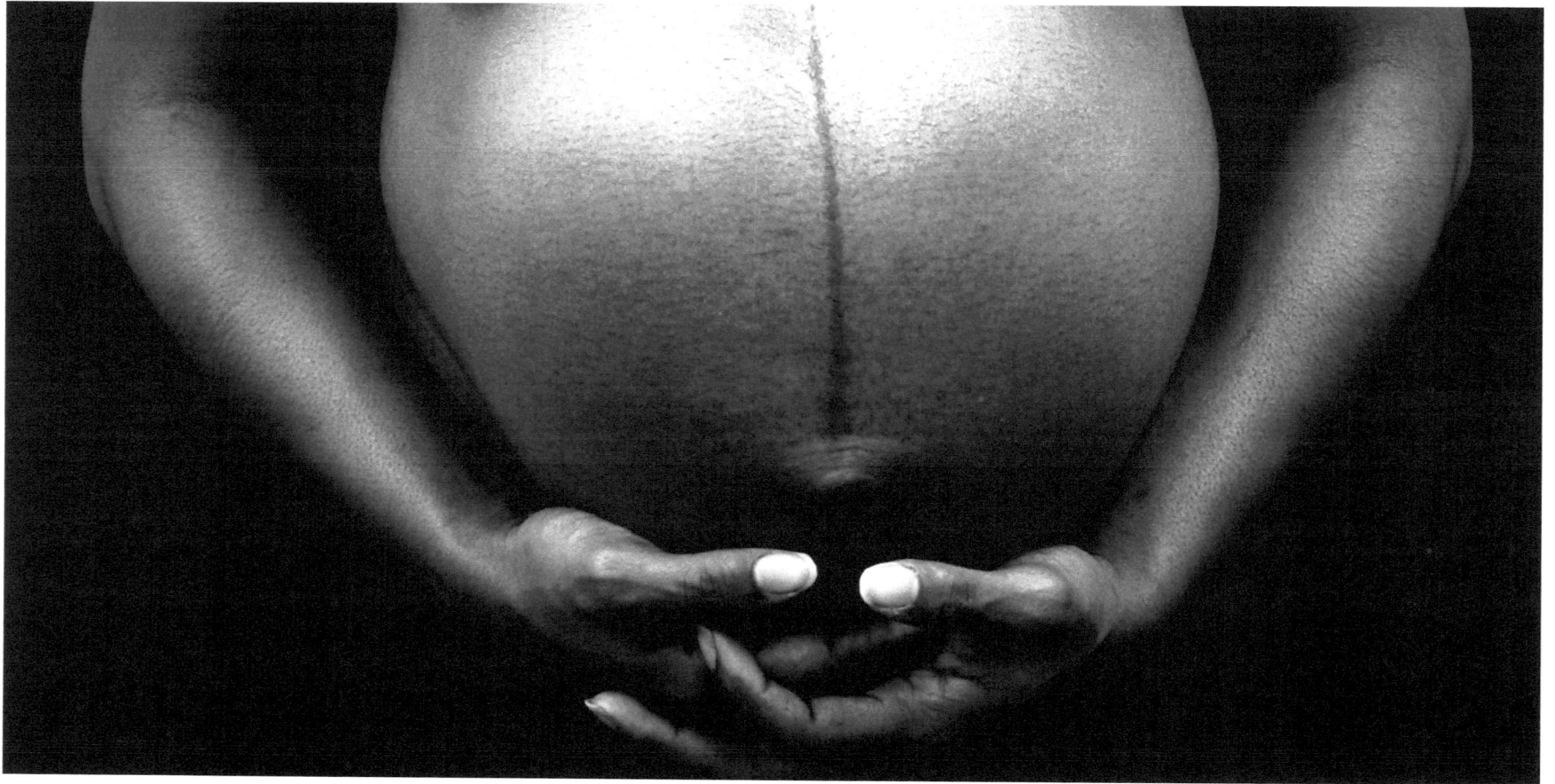

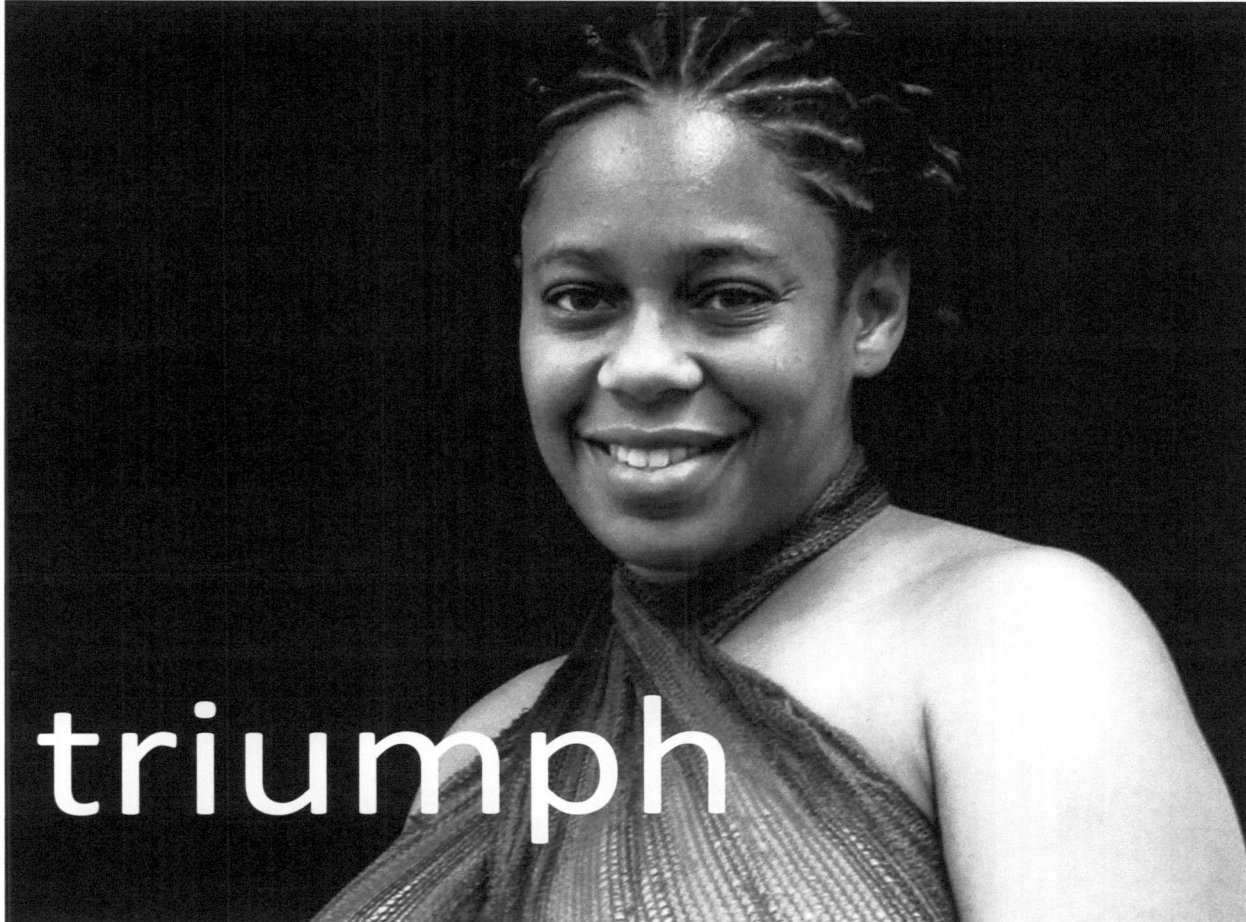

triumph

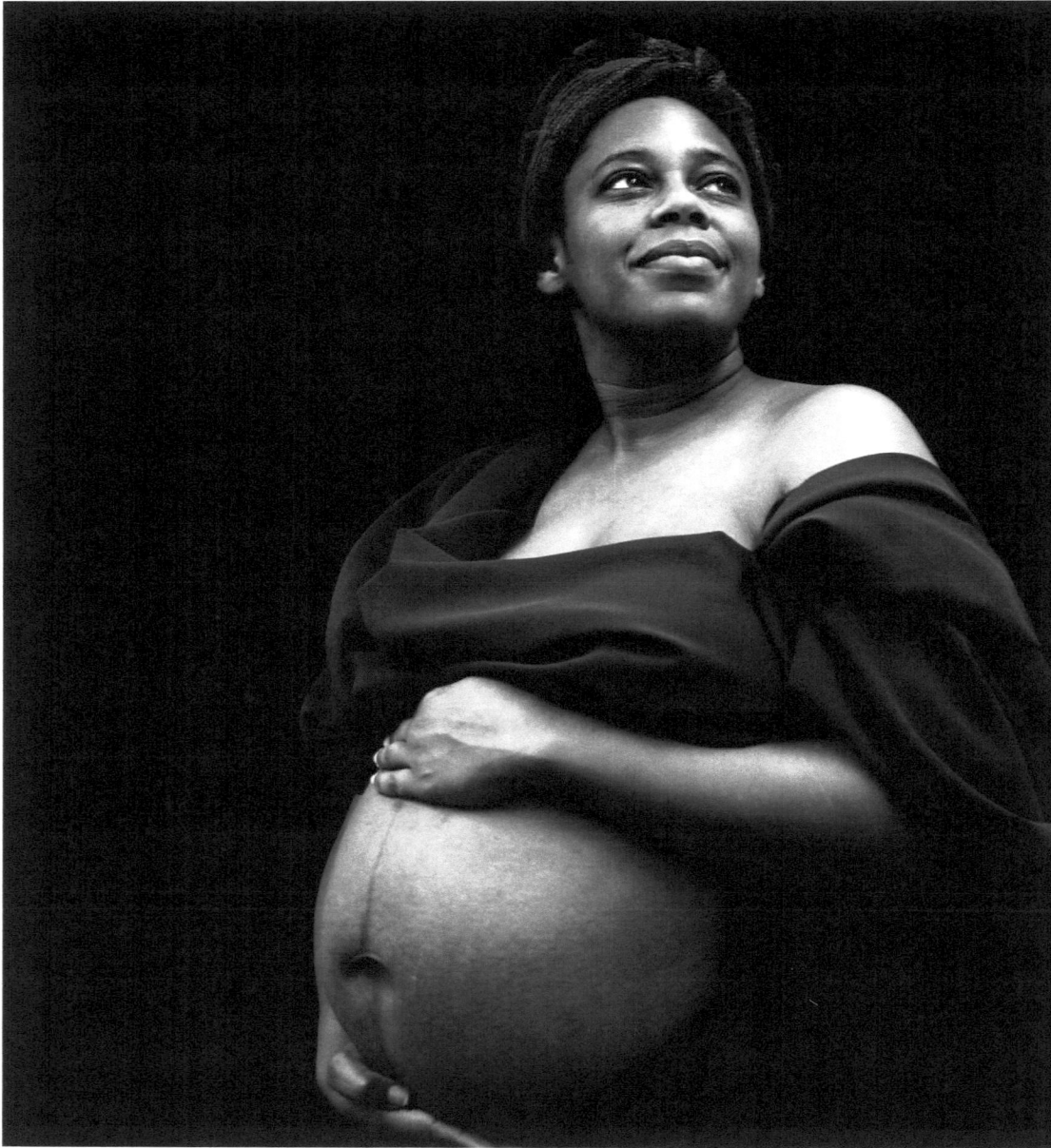

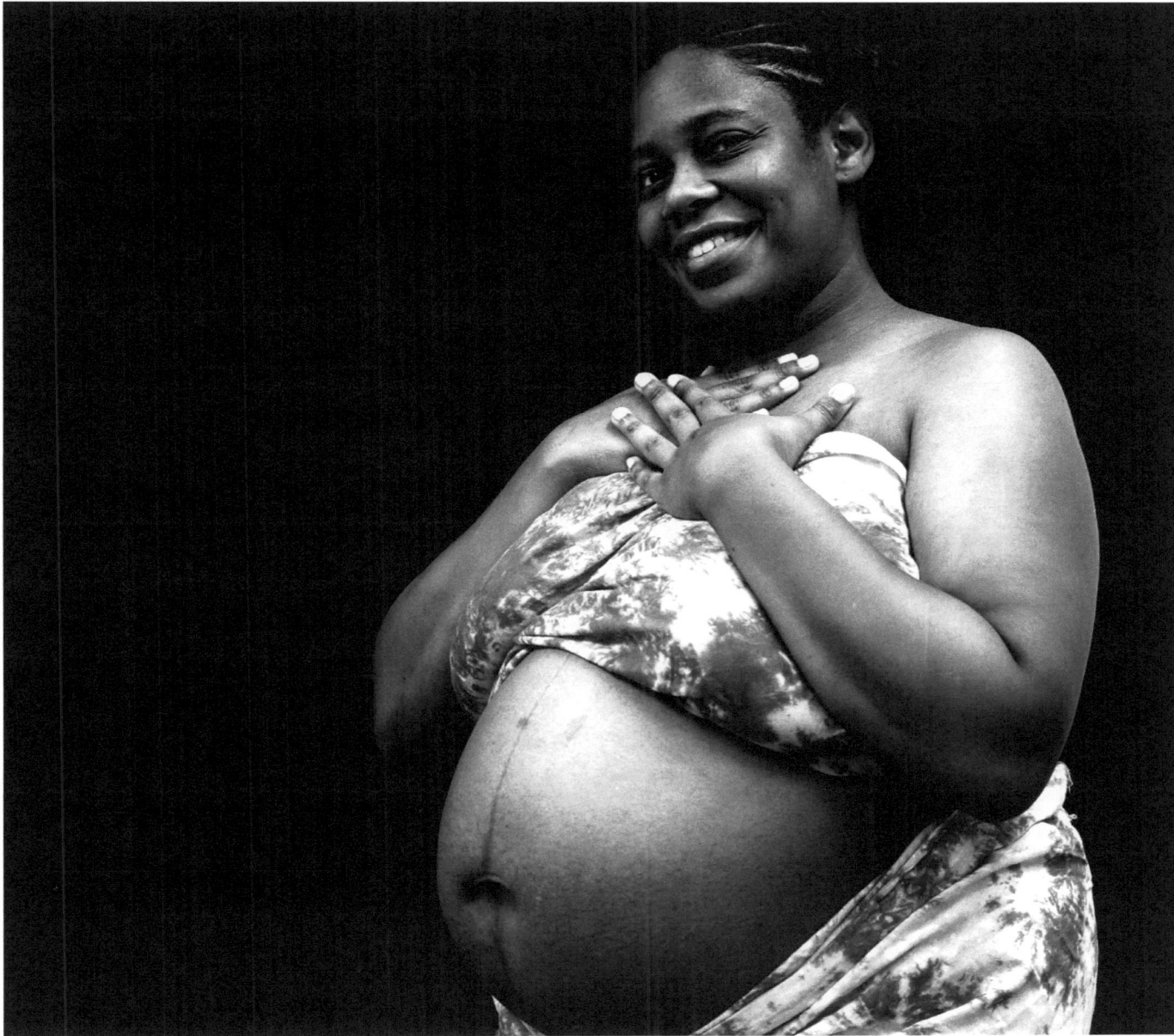

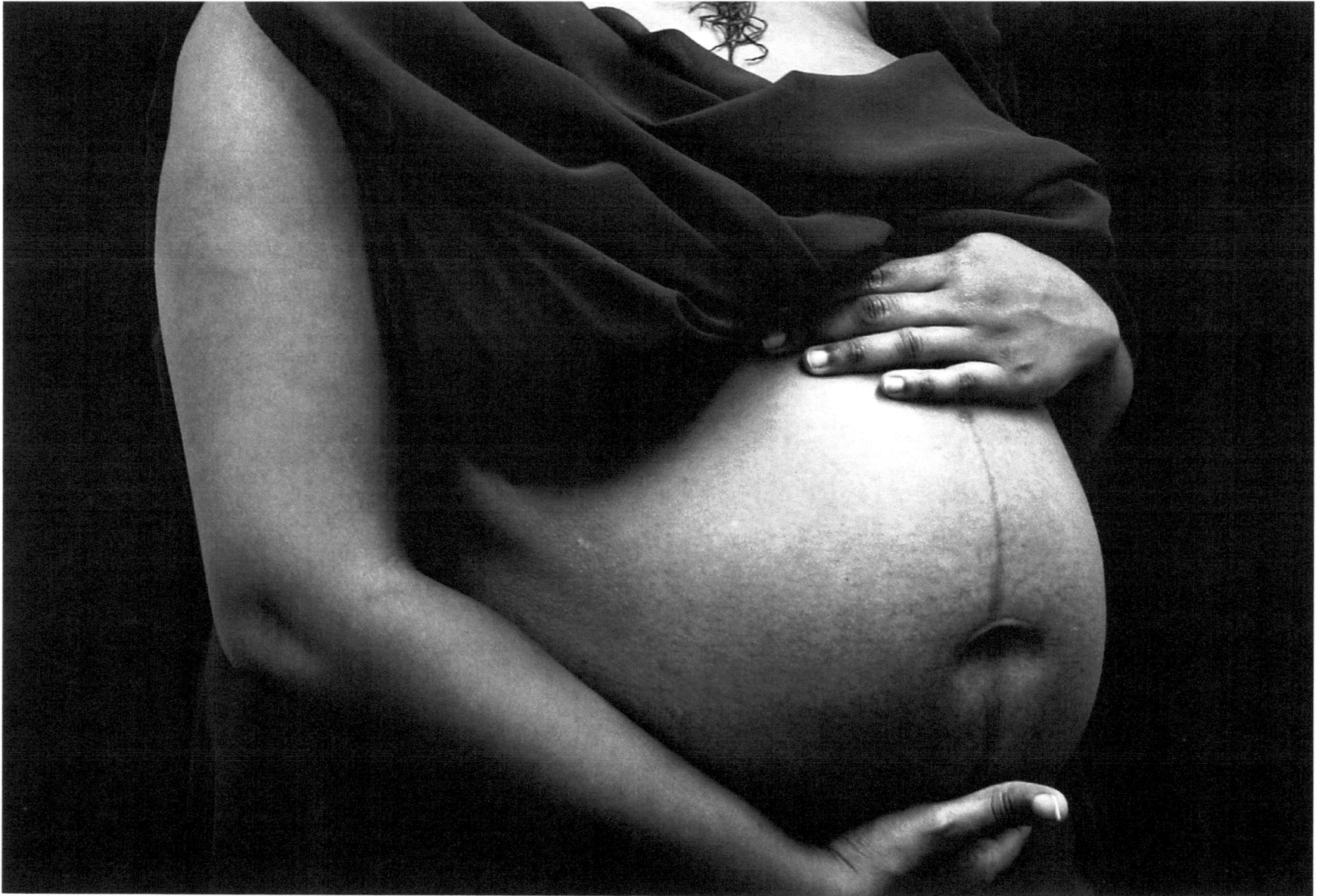

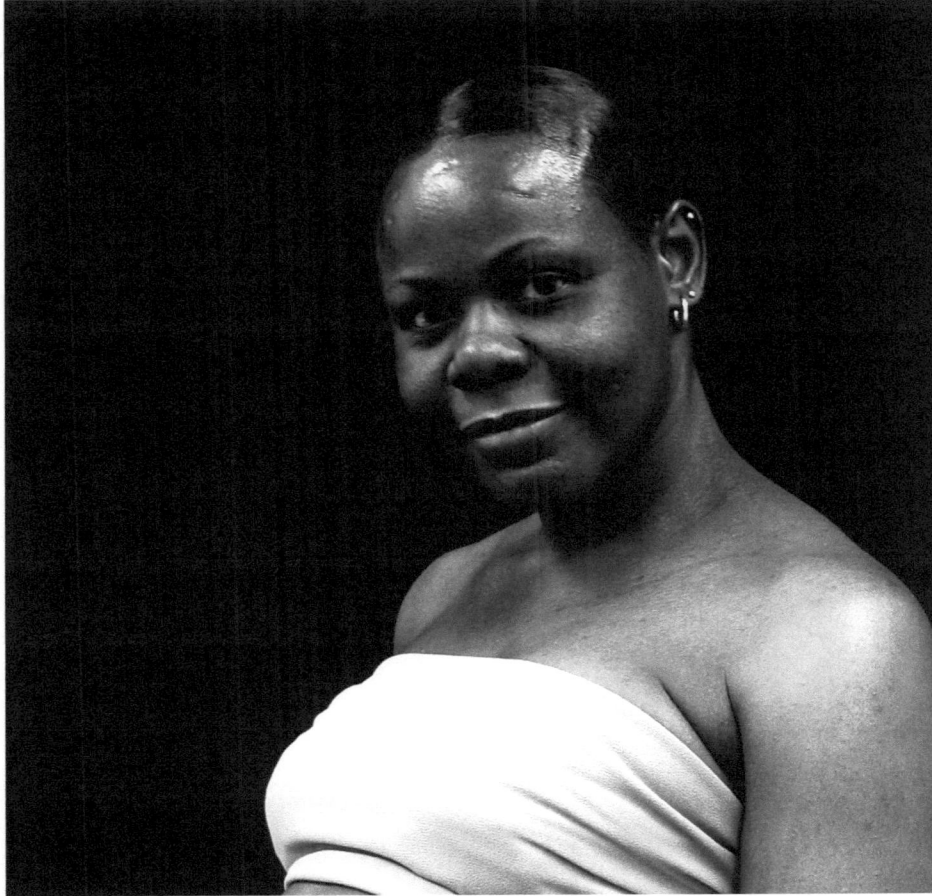

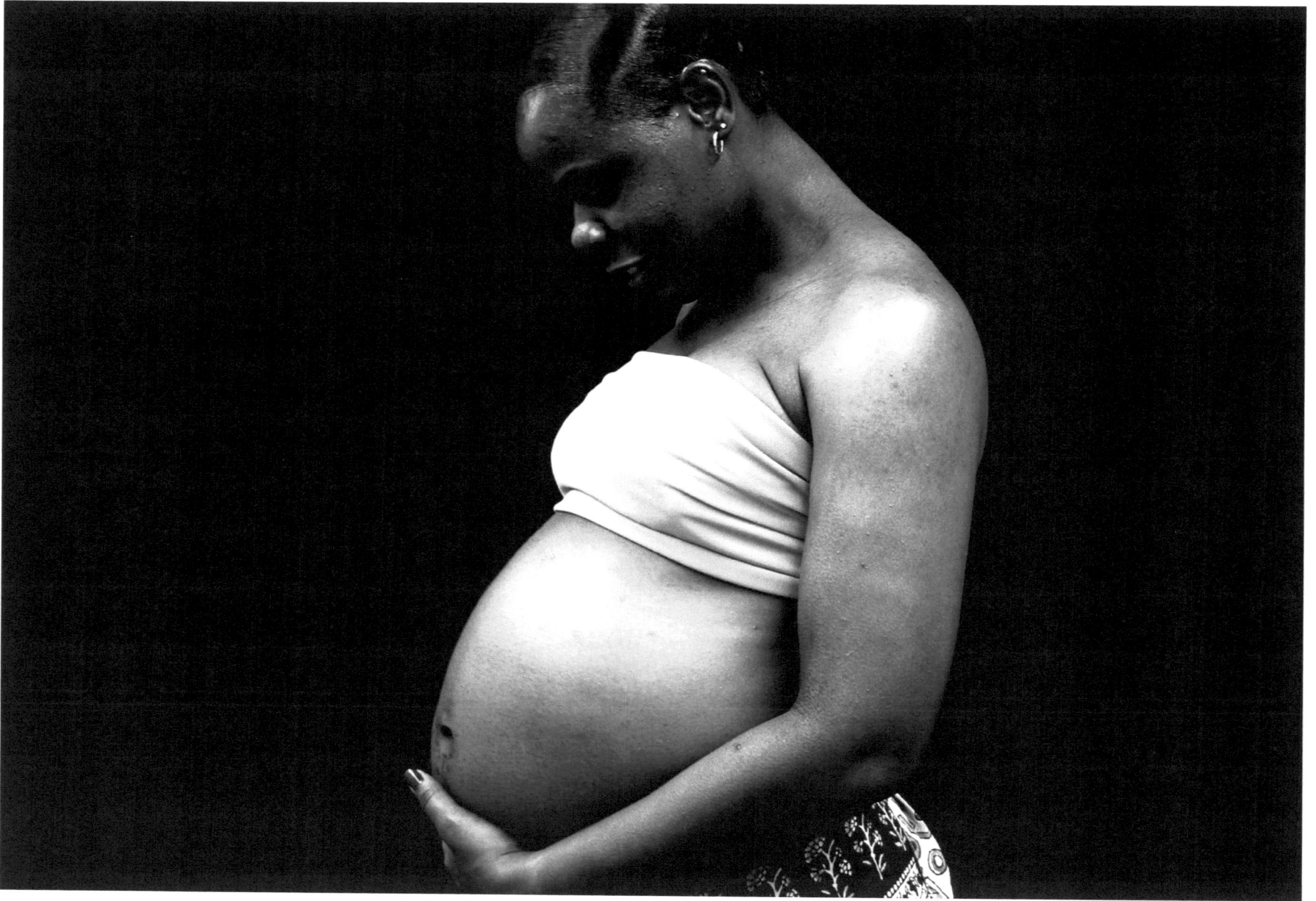

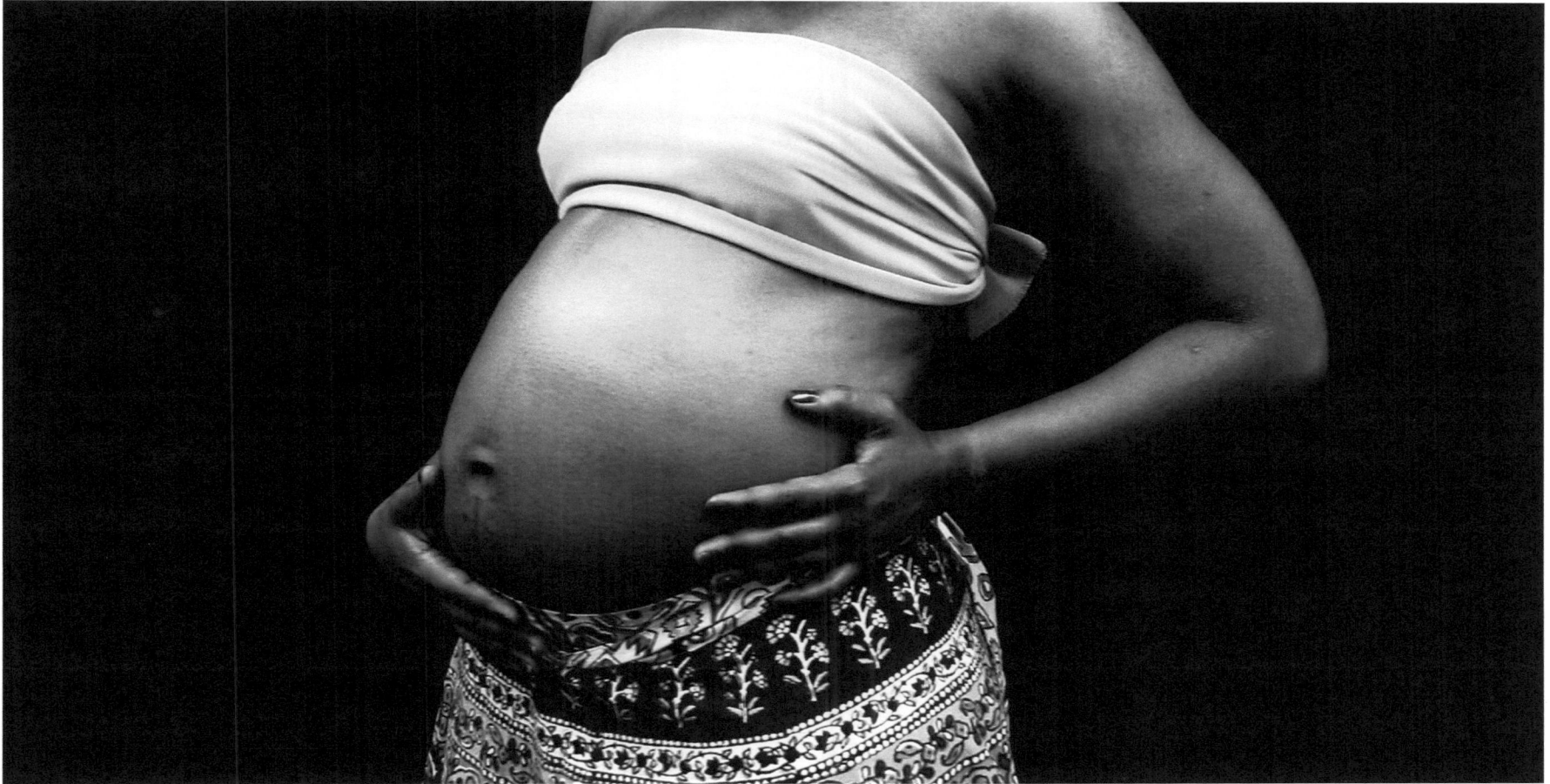

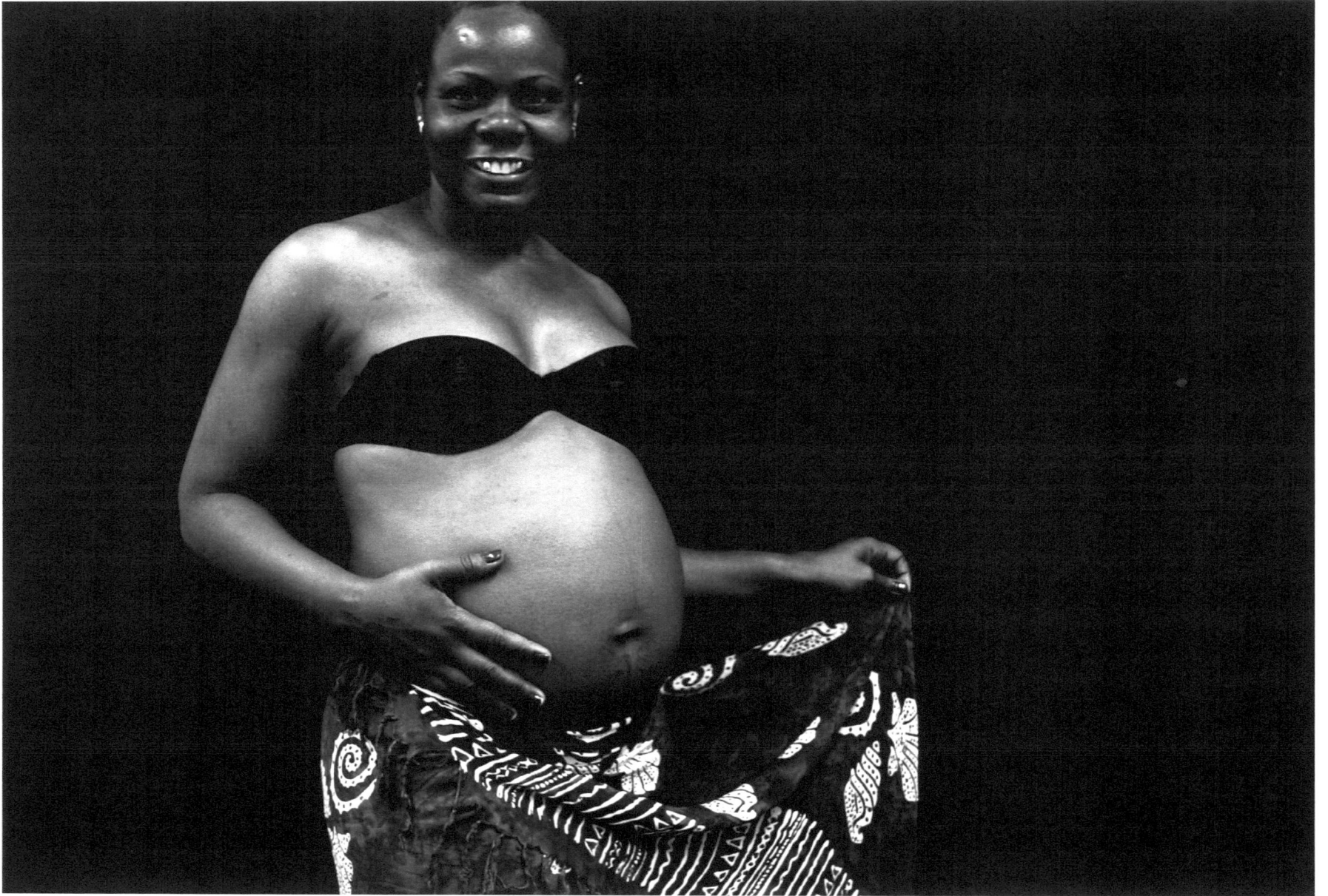

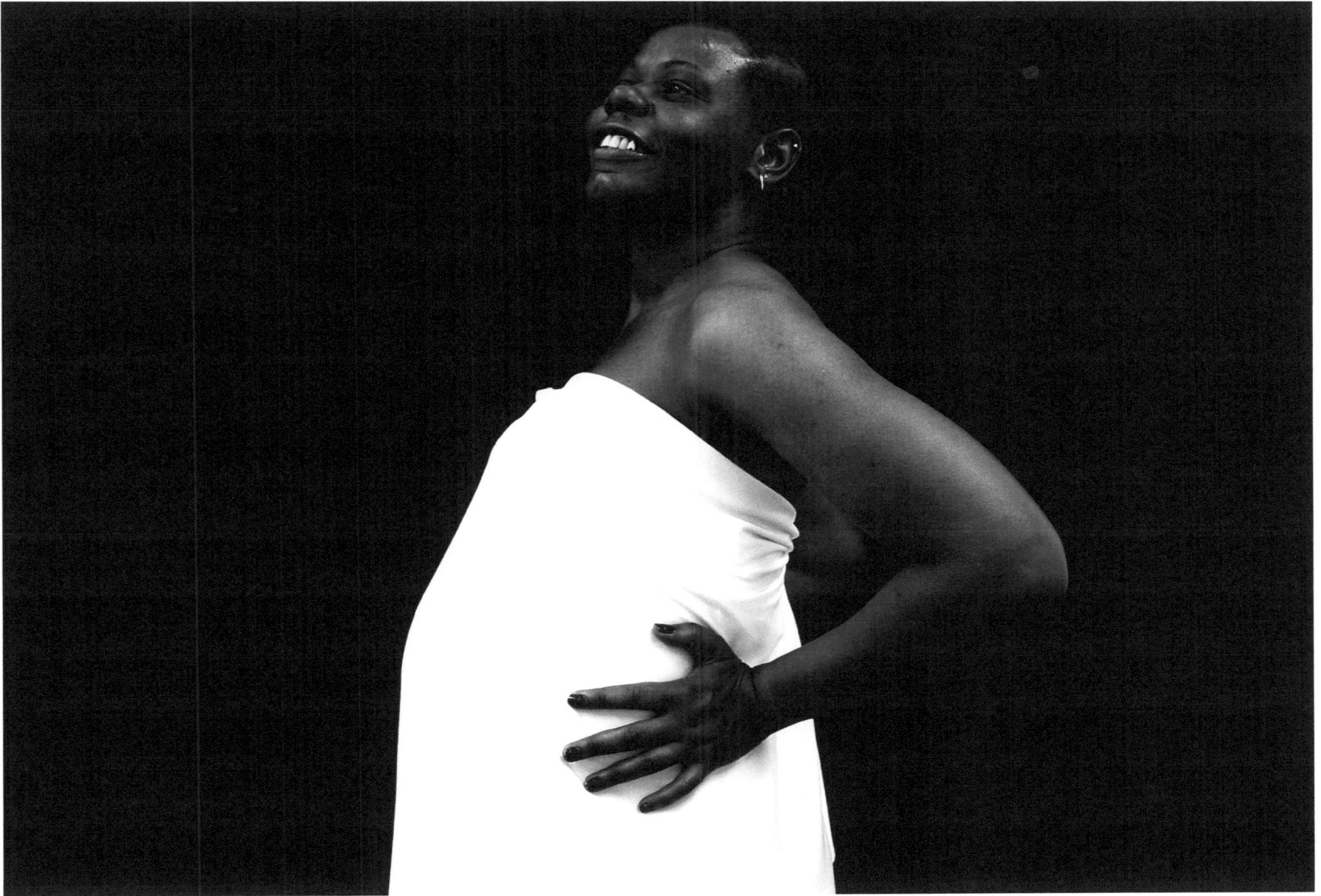

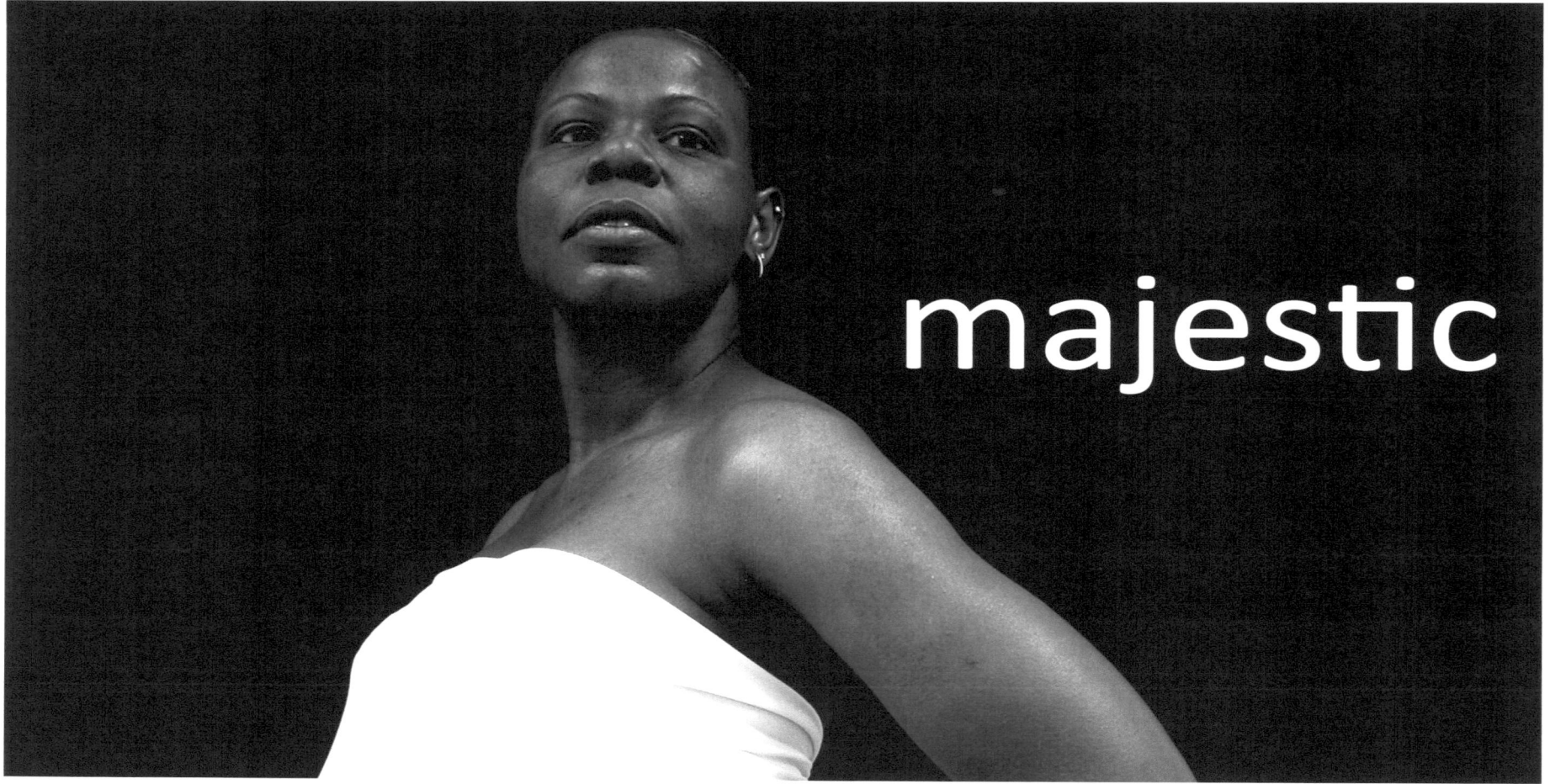

majestic

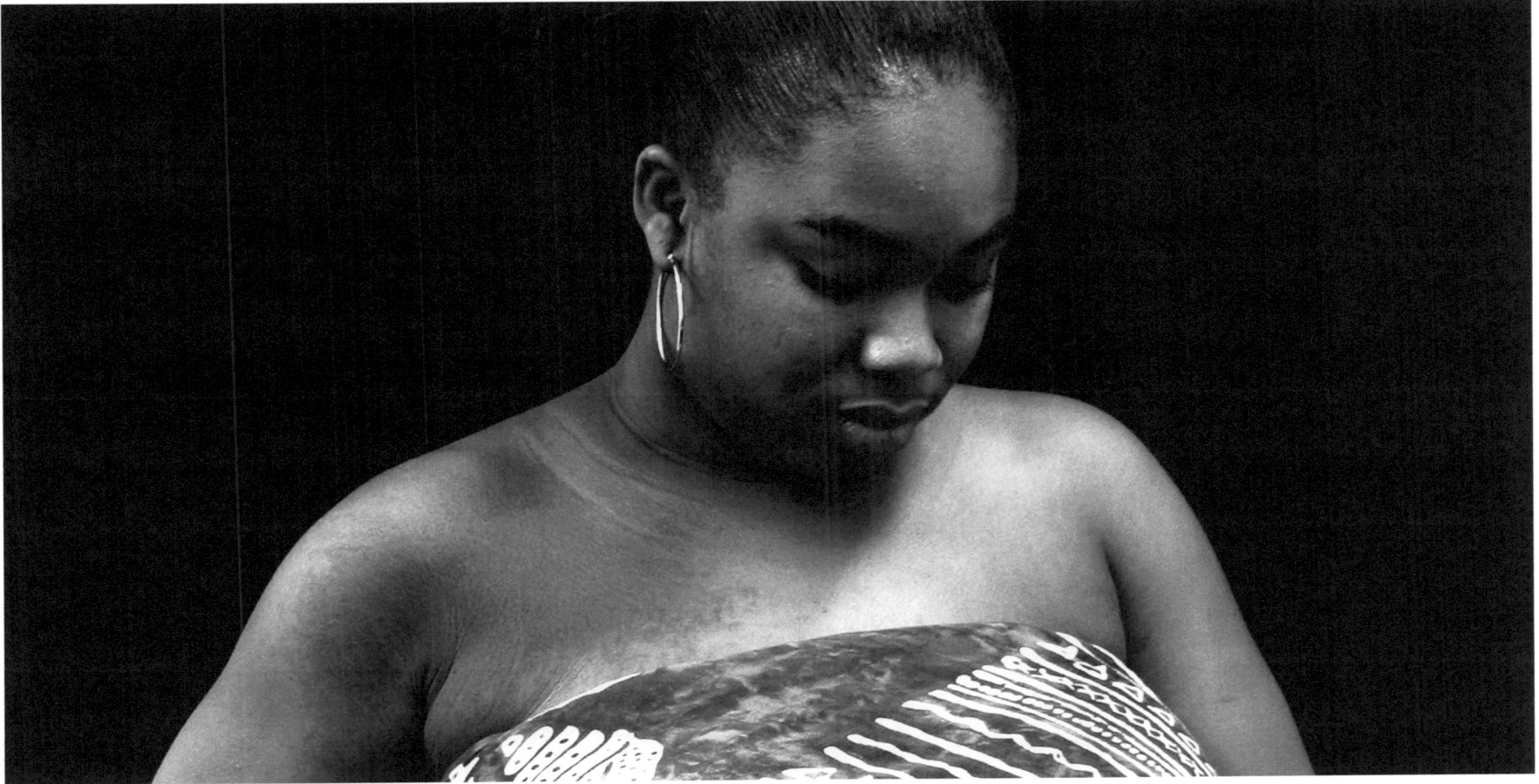

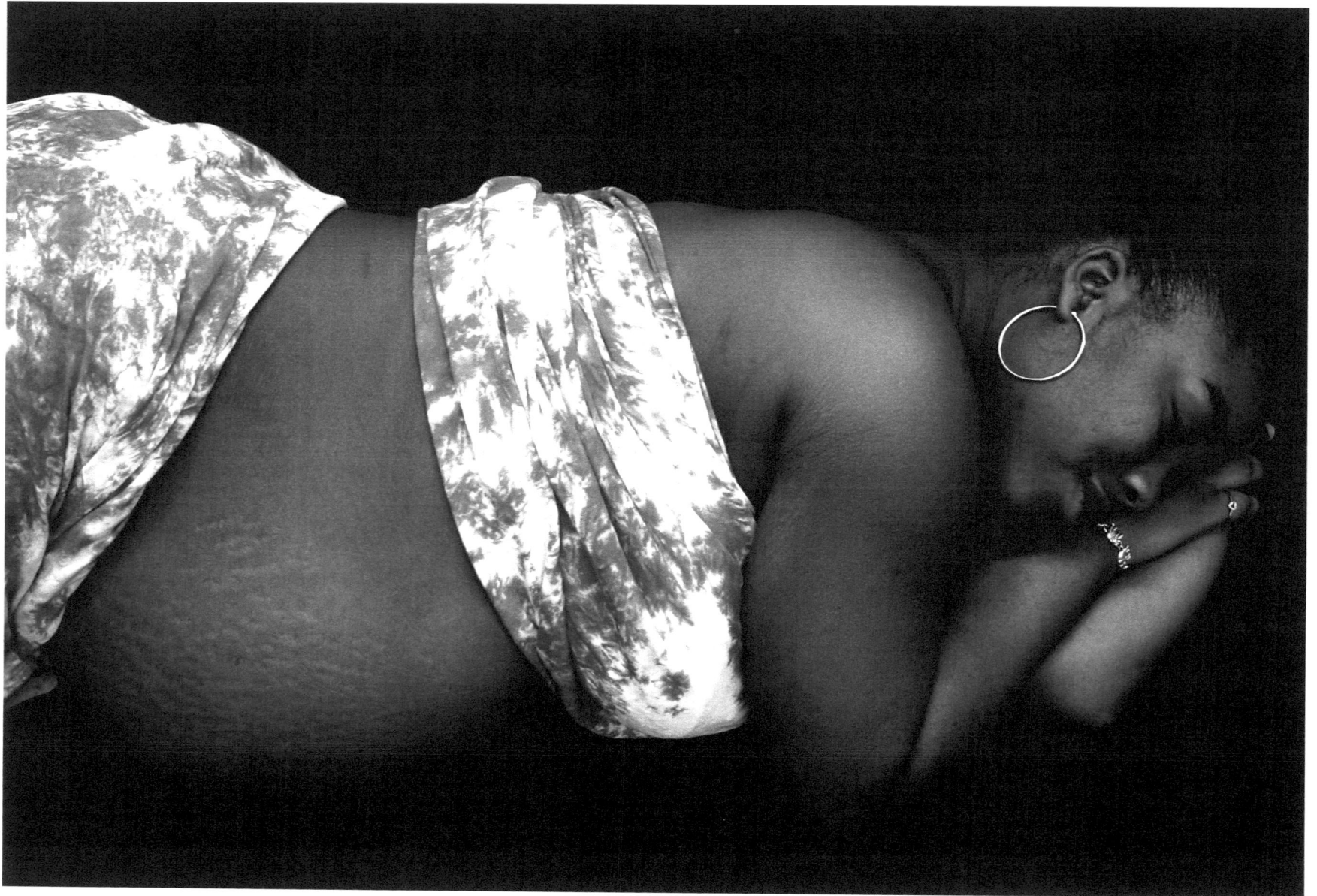

delight

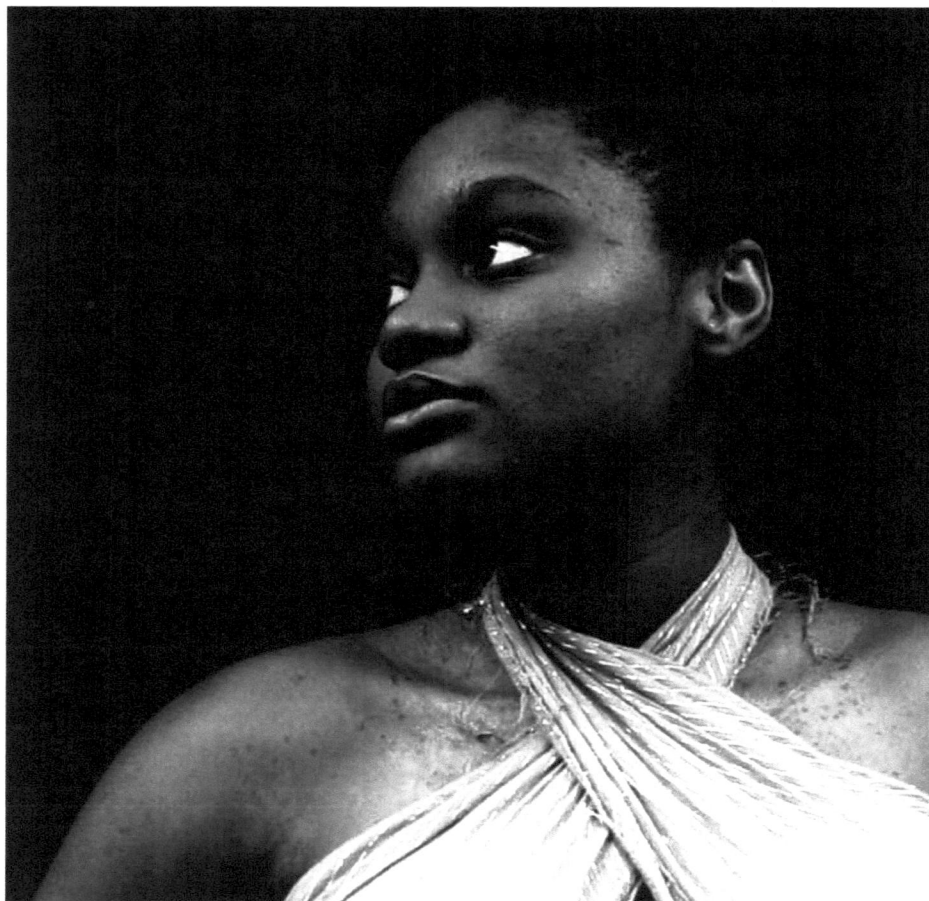

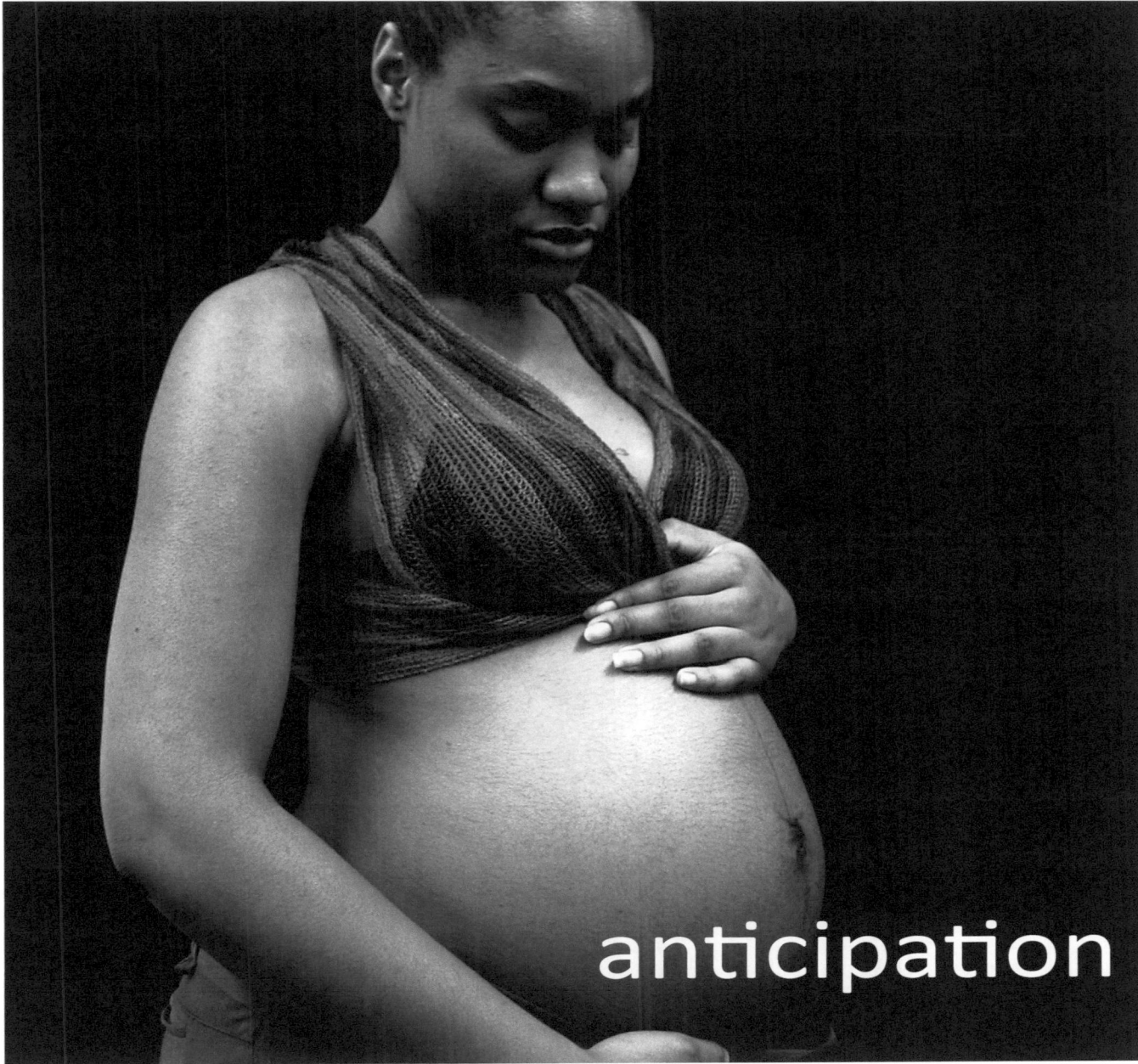

anticipation

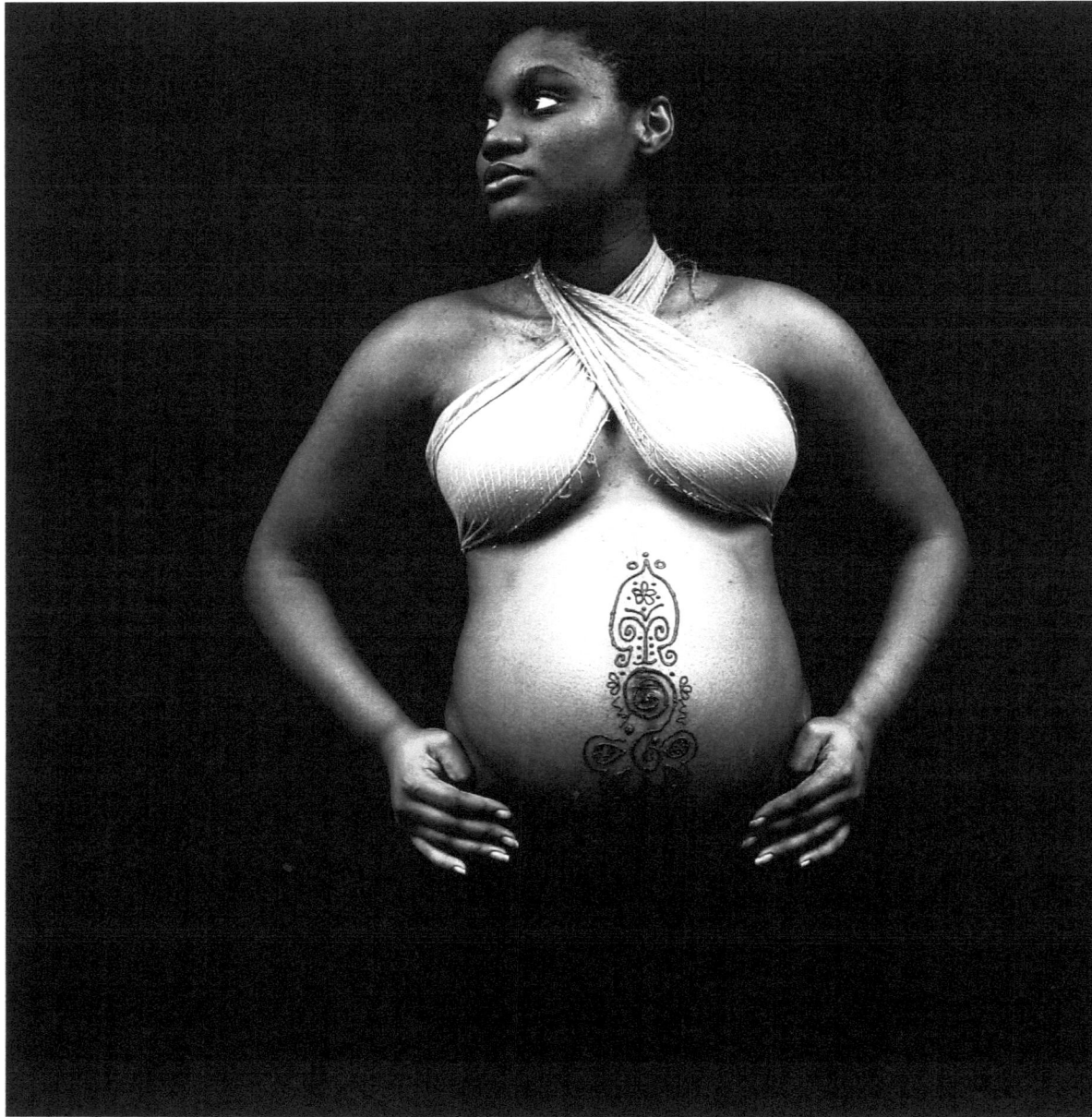

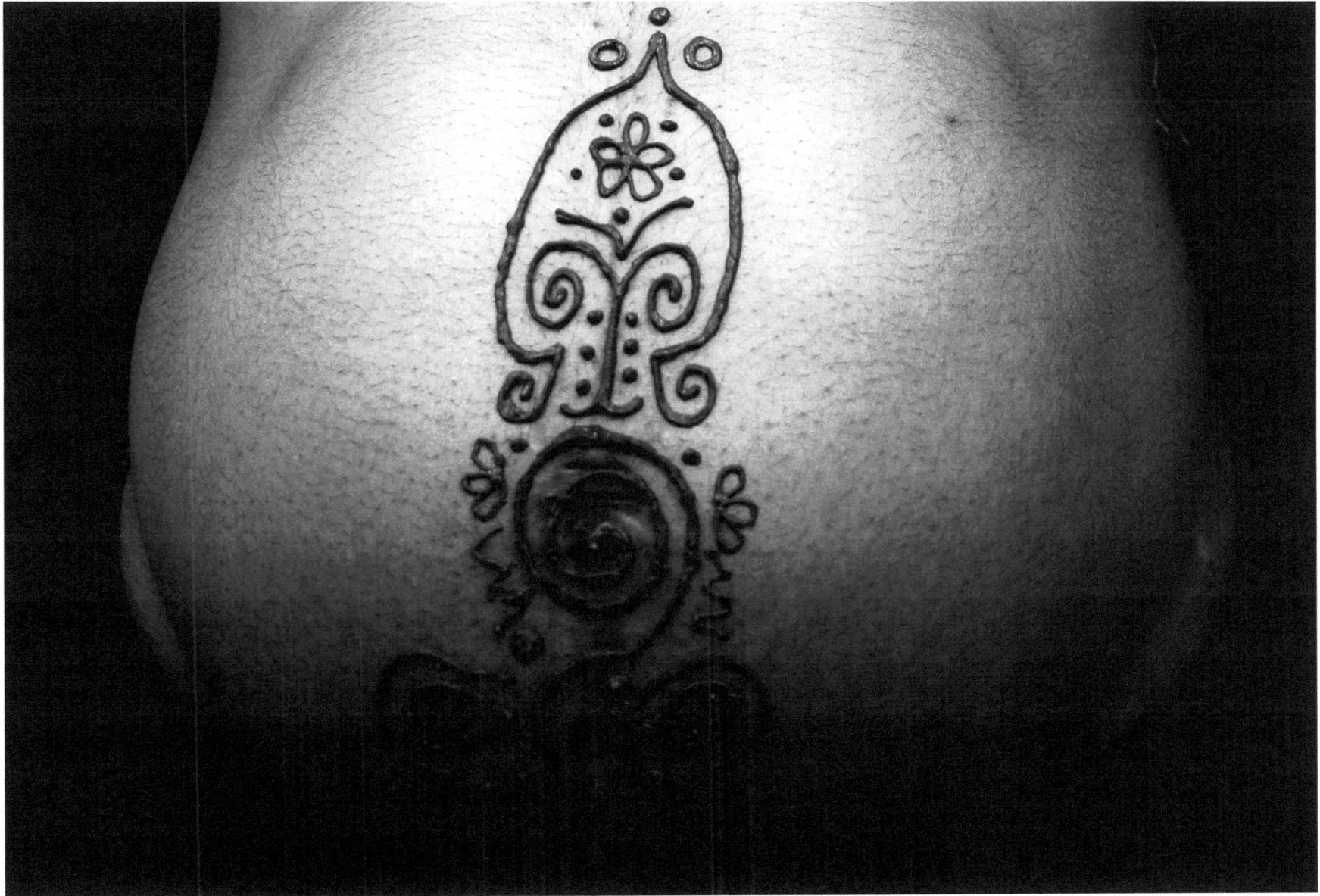

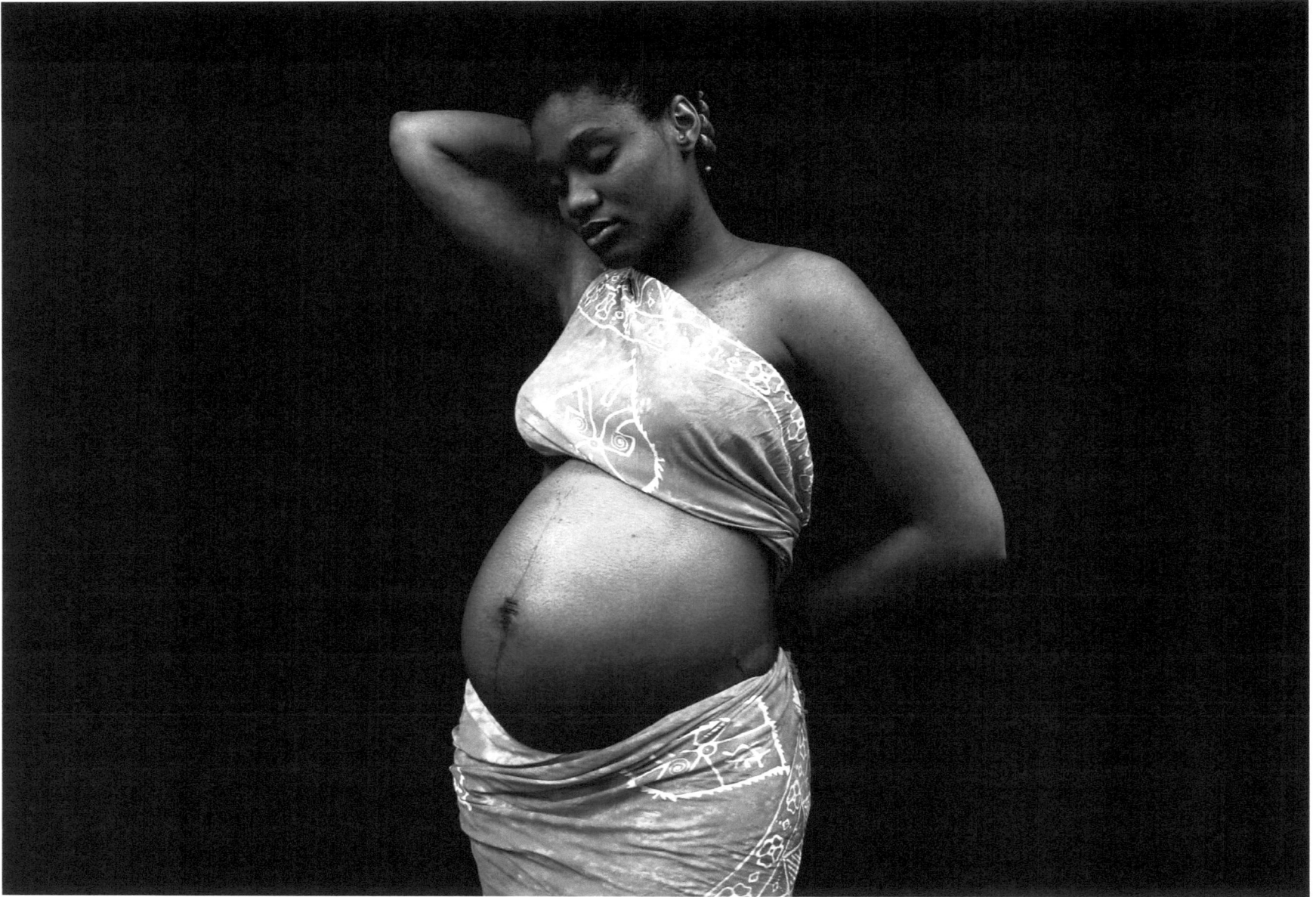

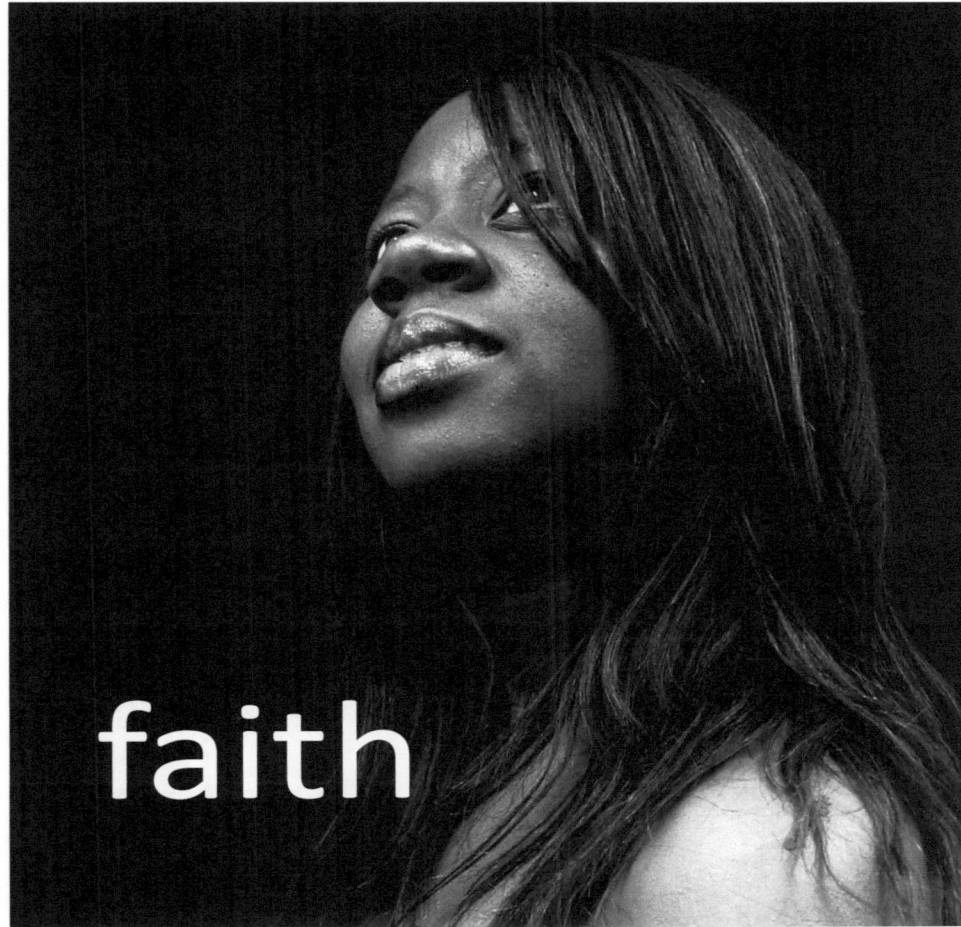

faith

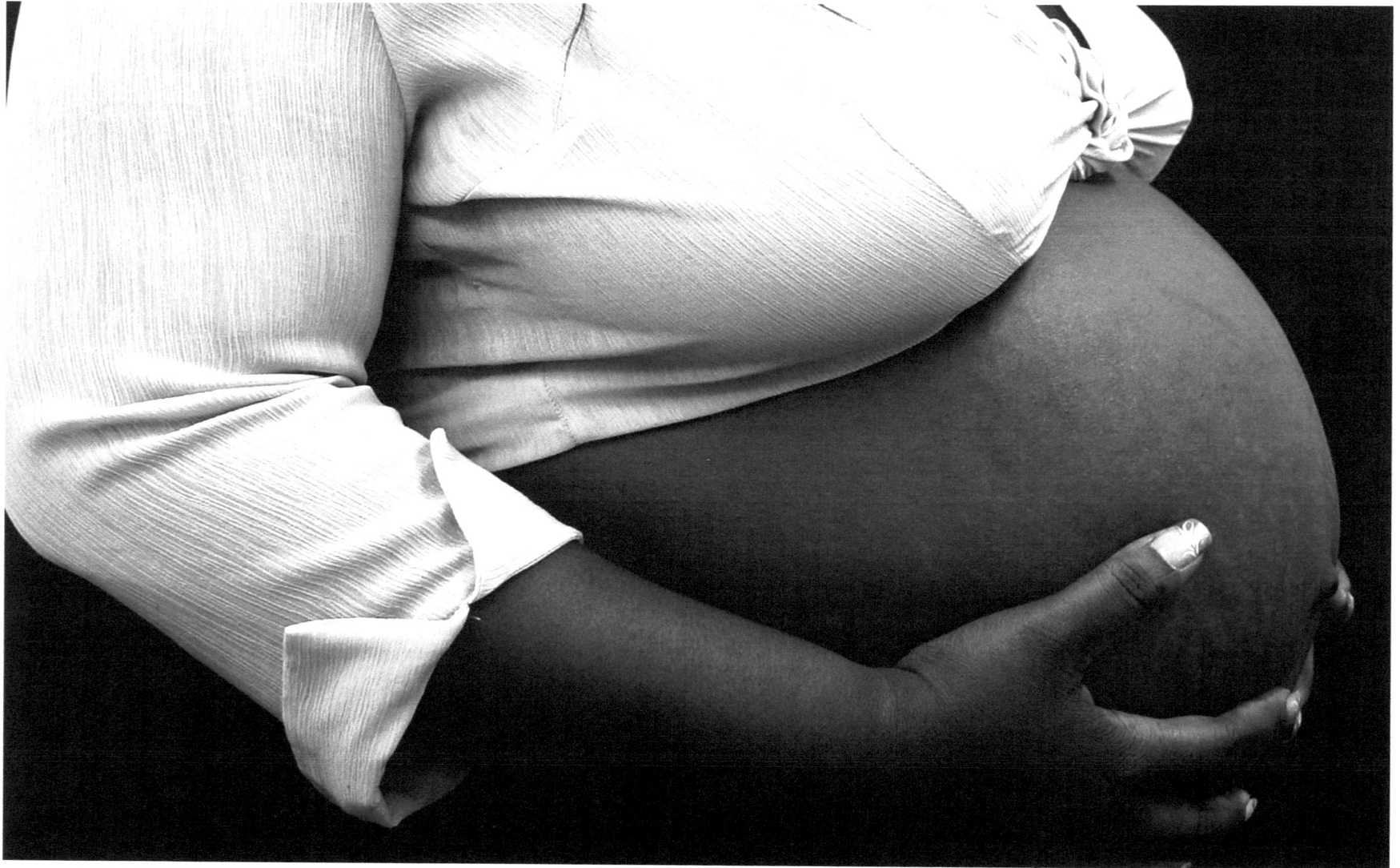

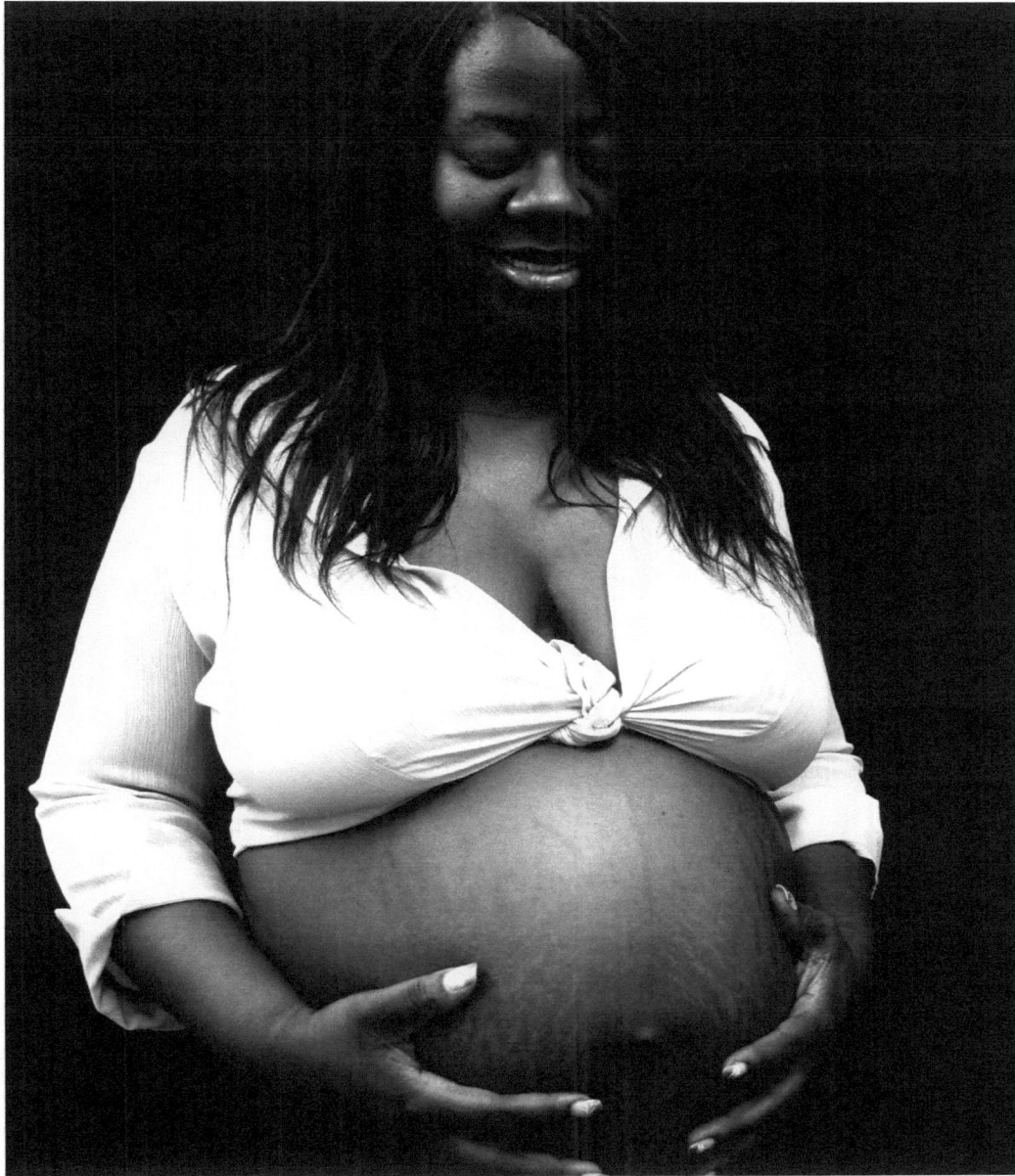

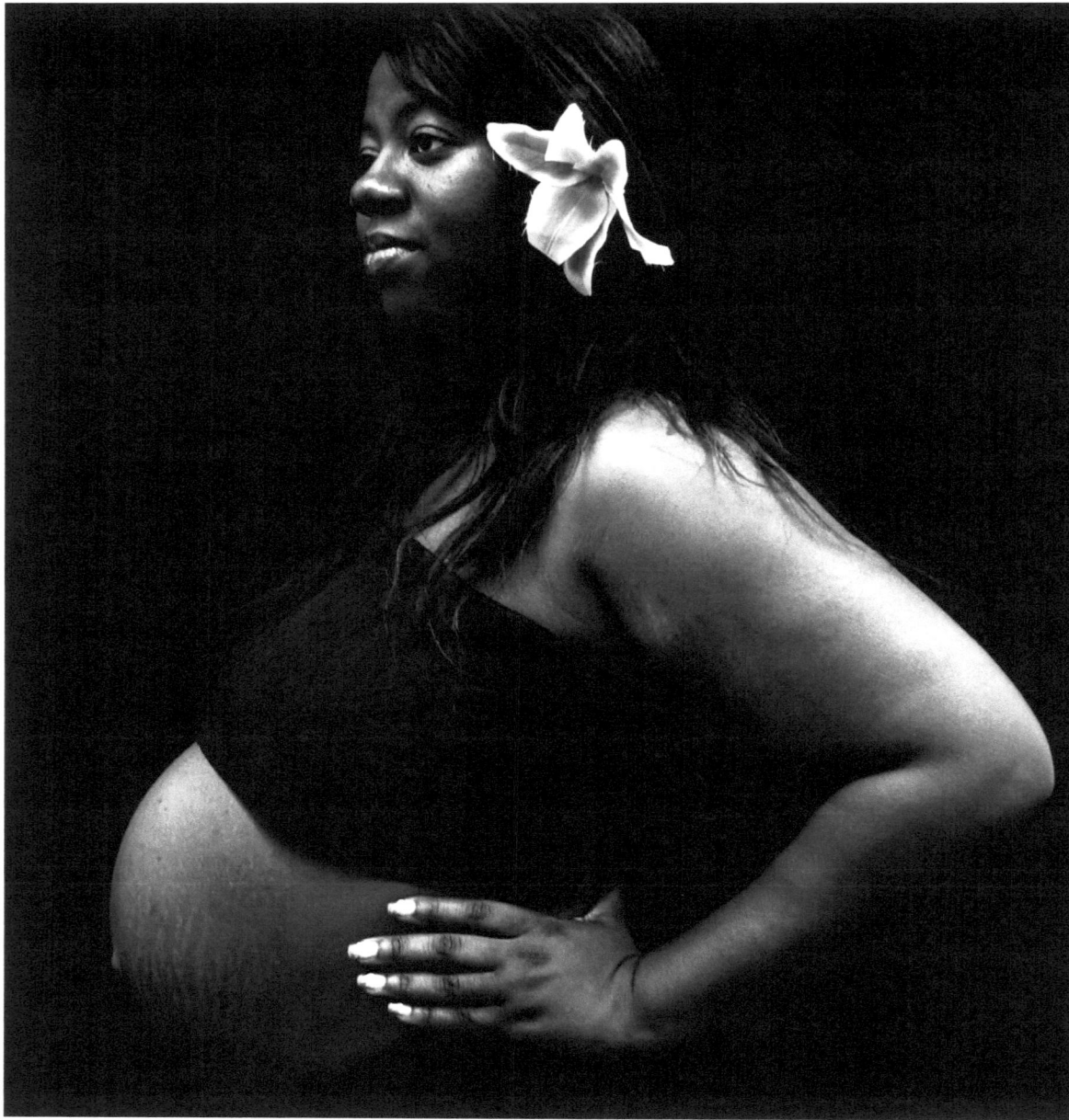

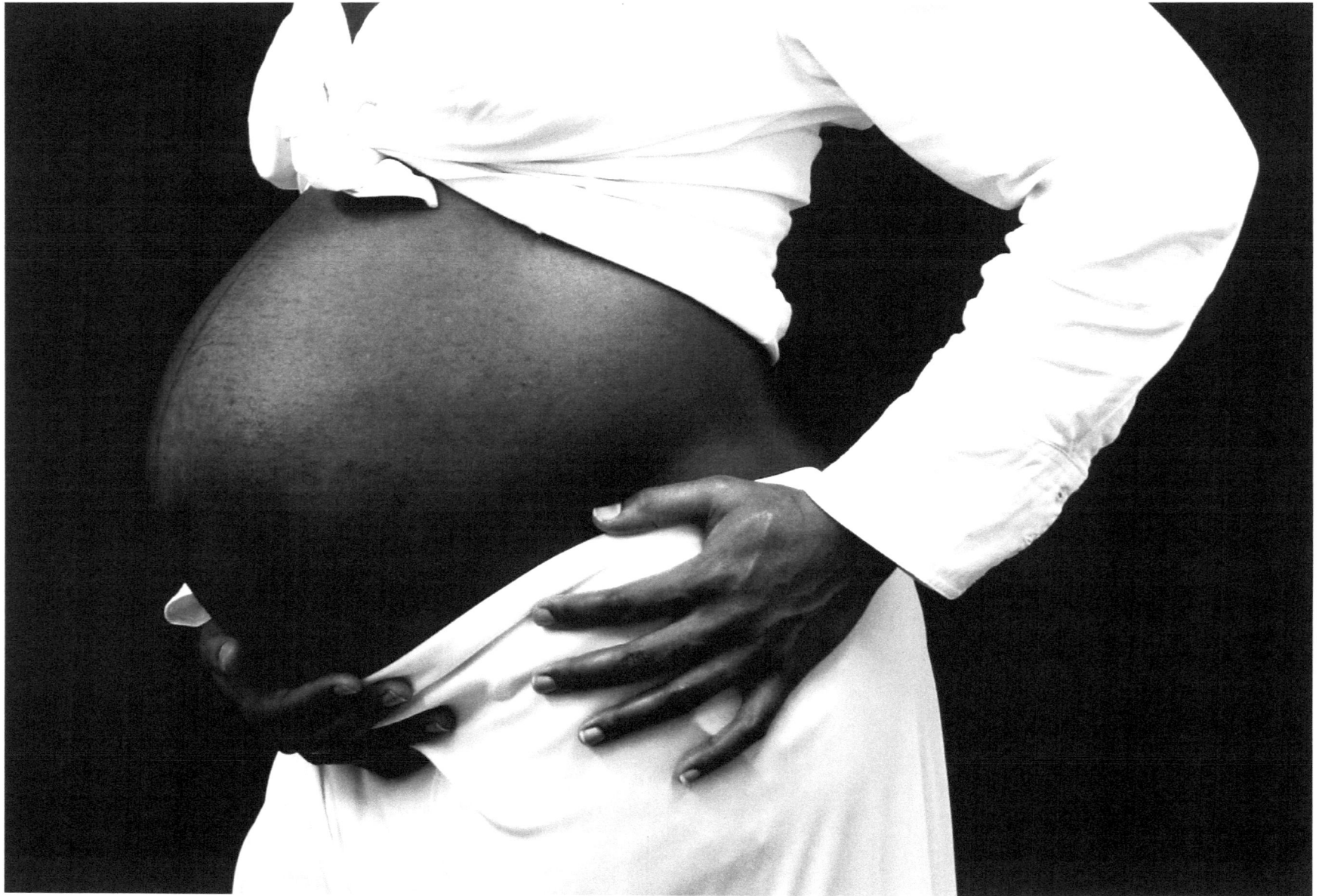

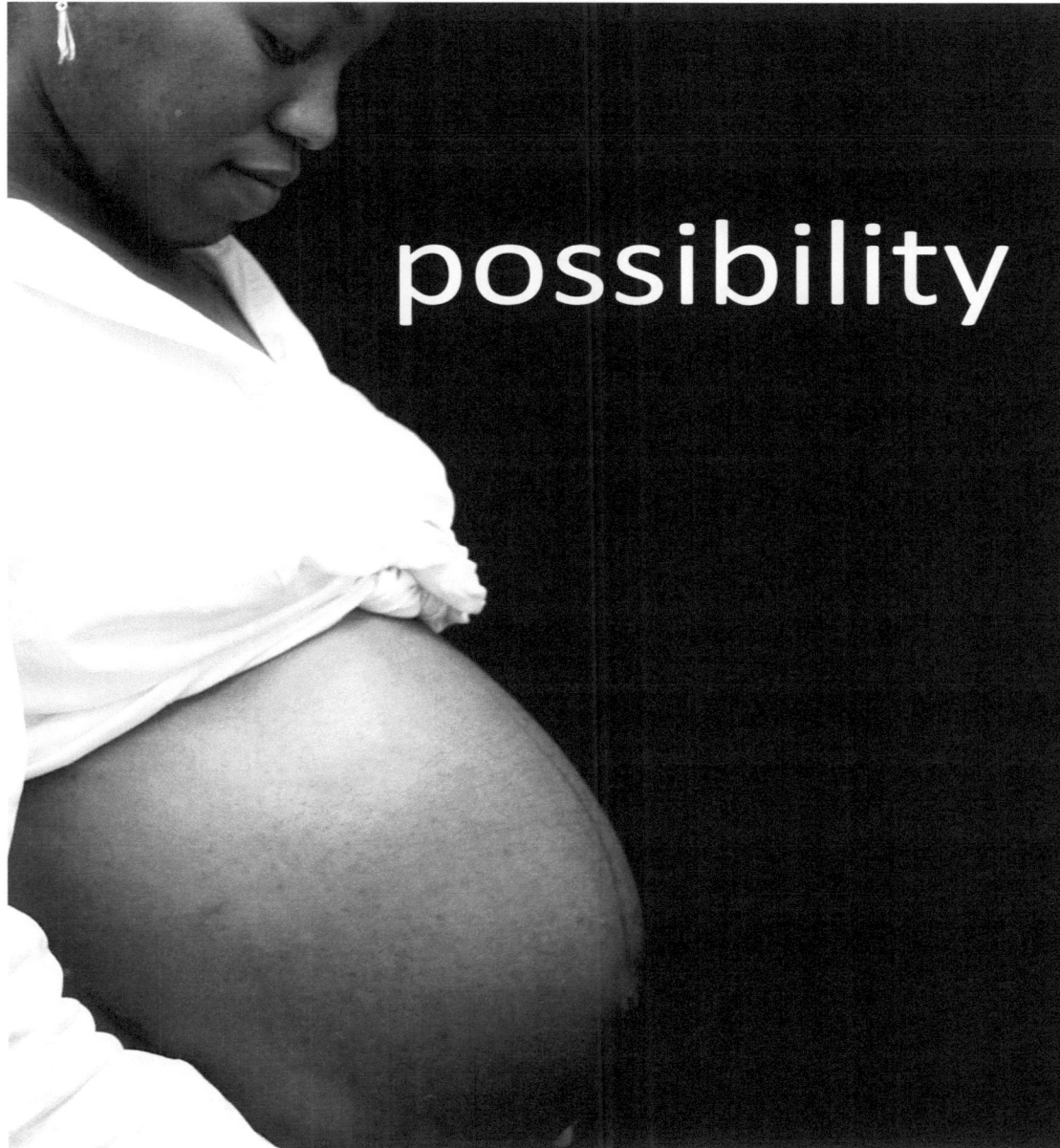

possibility

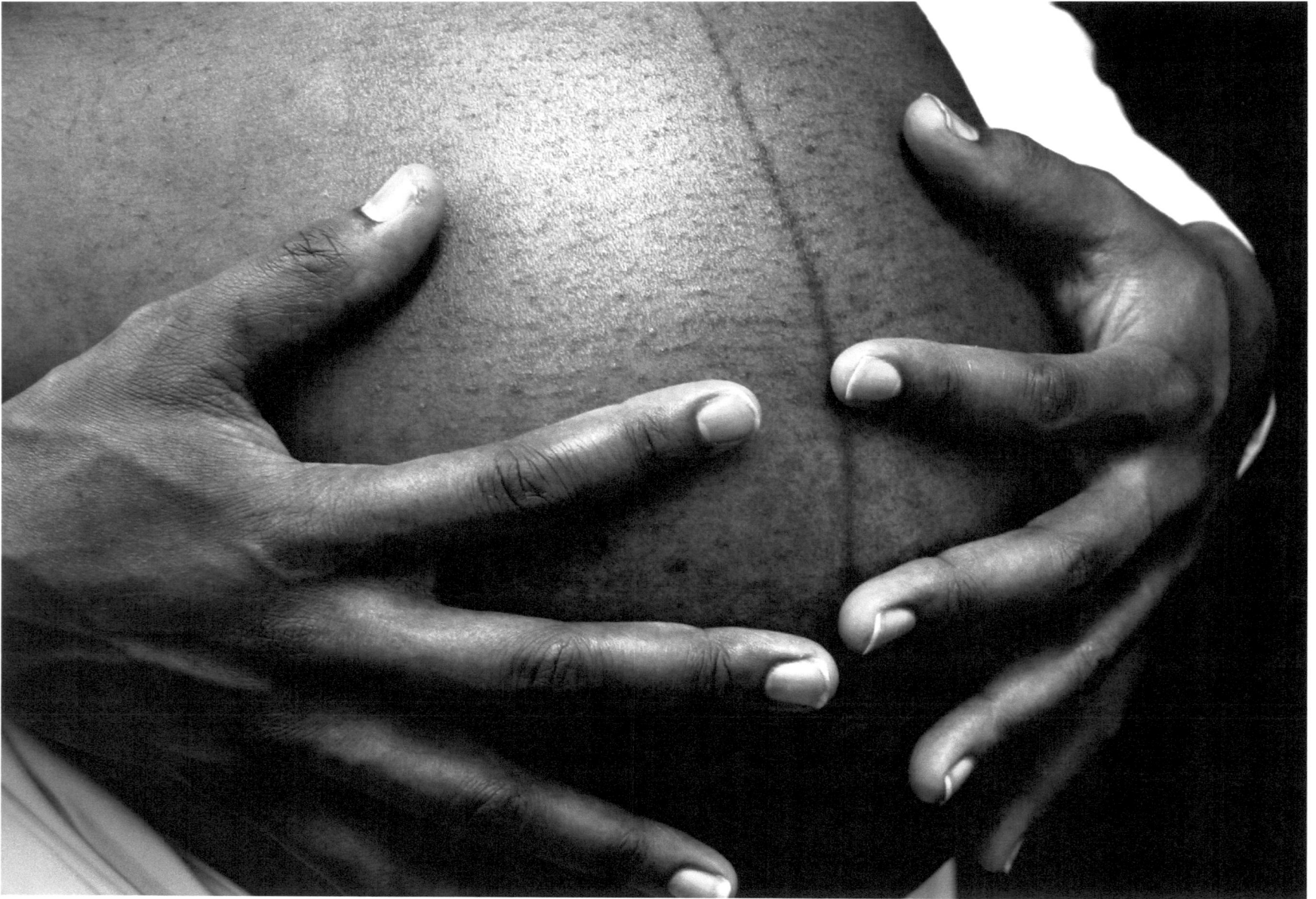

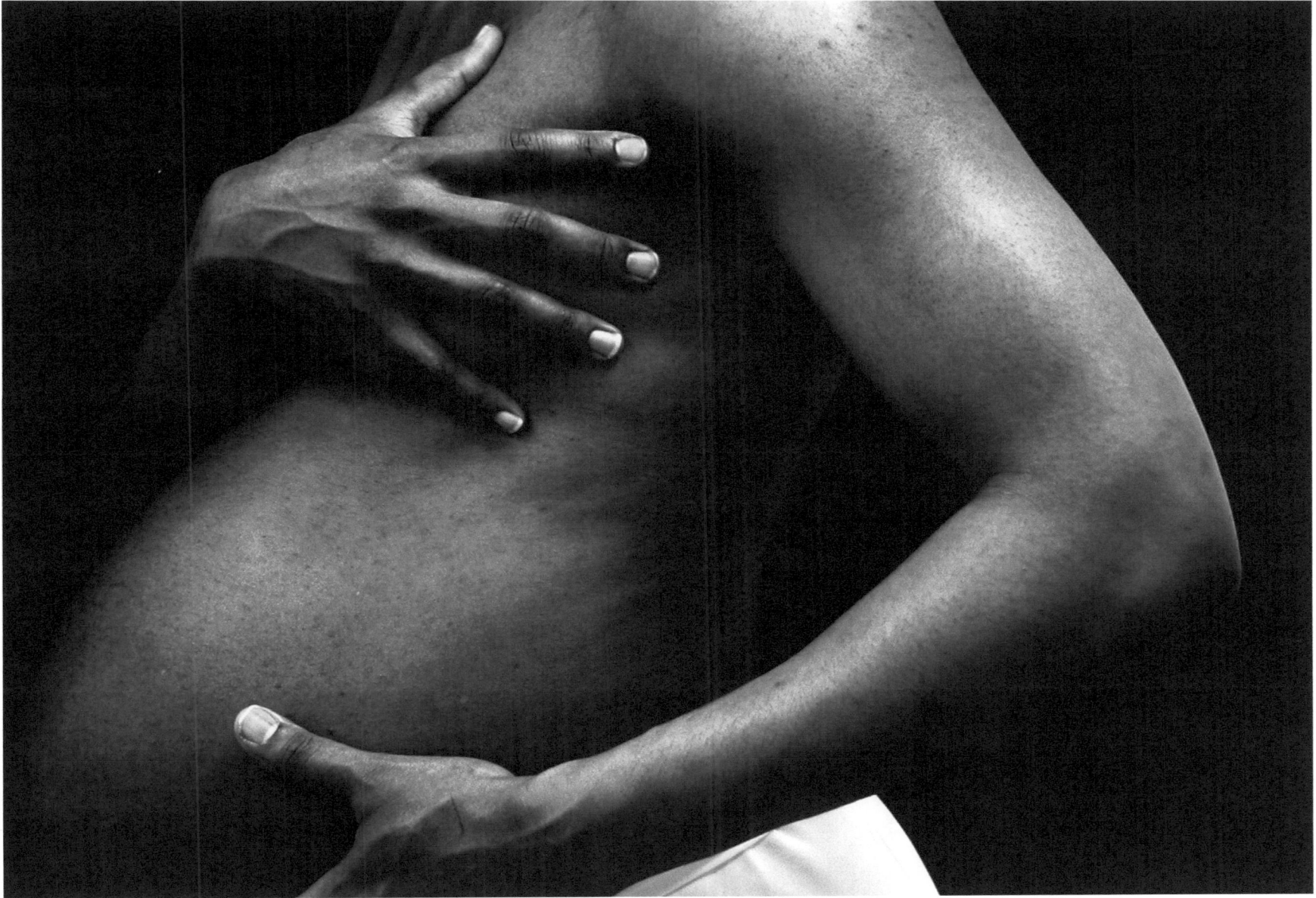

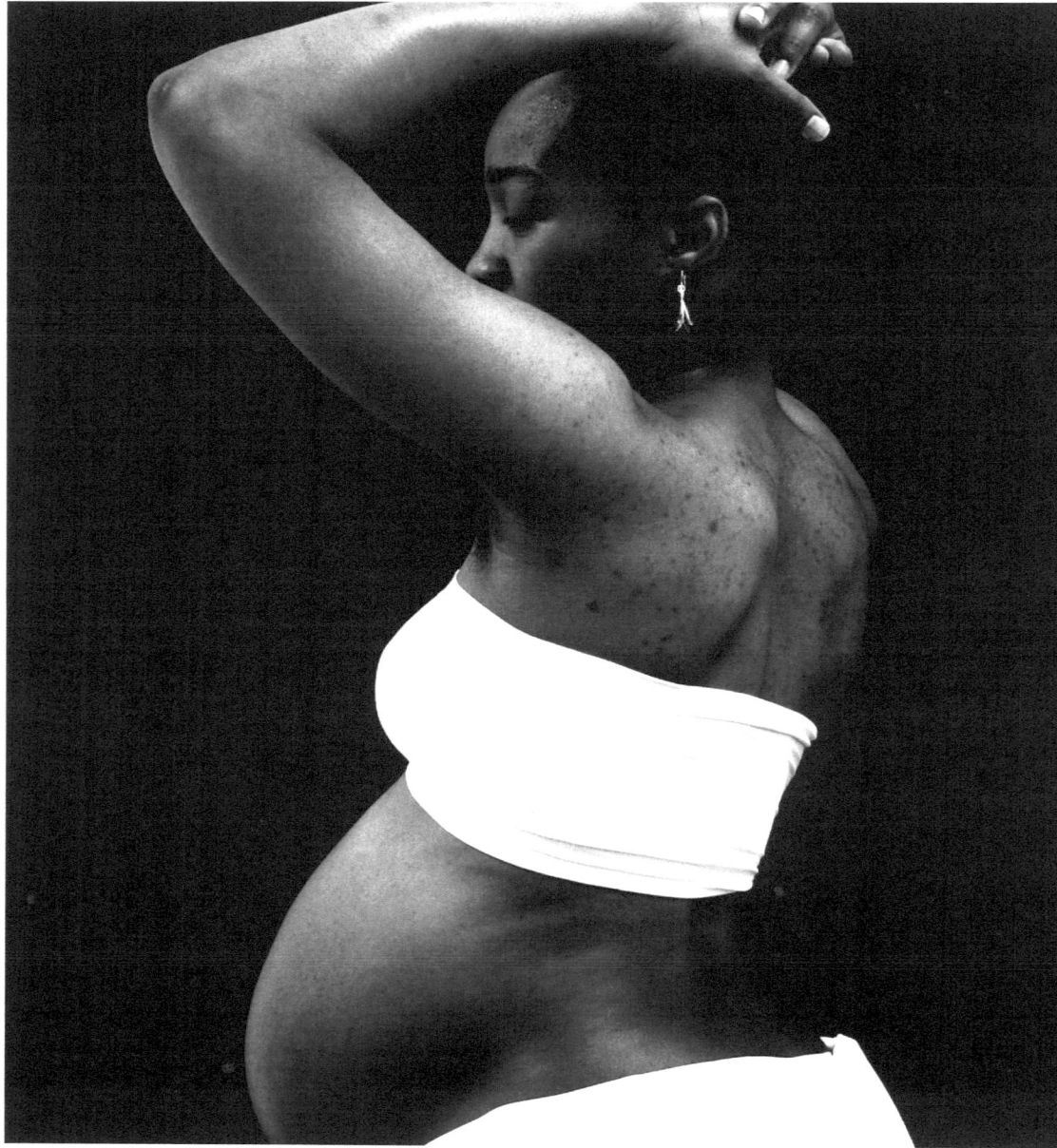

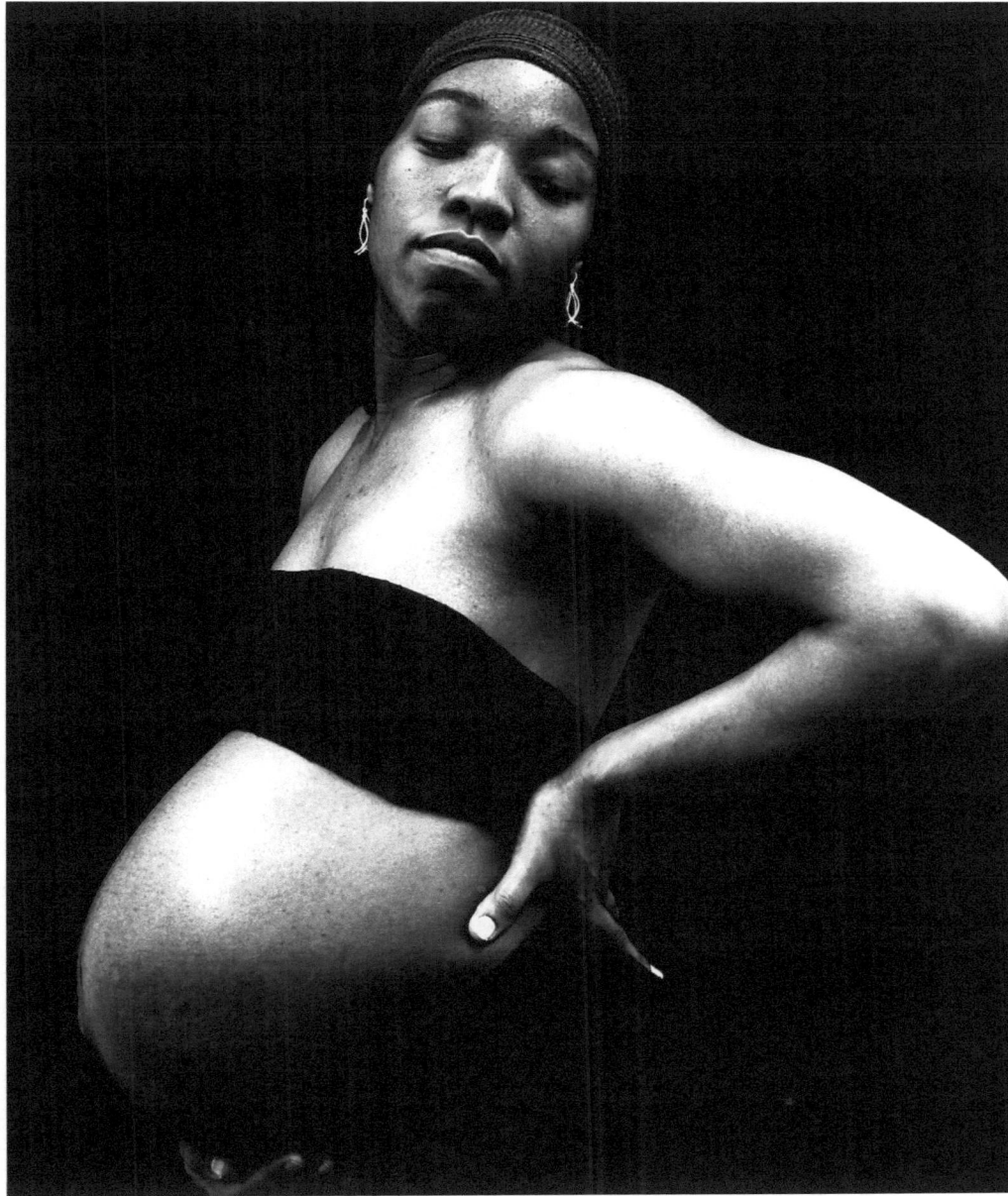

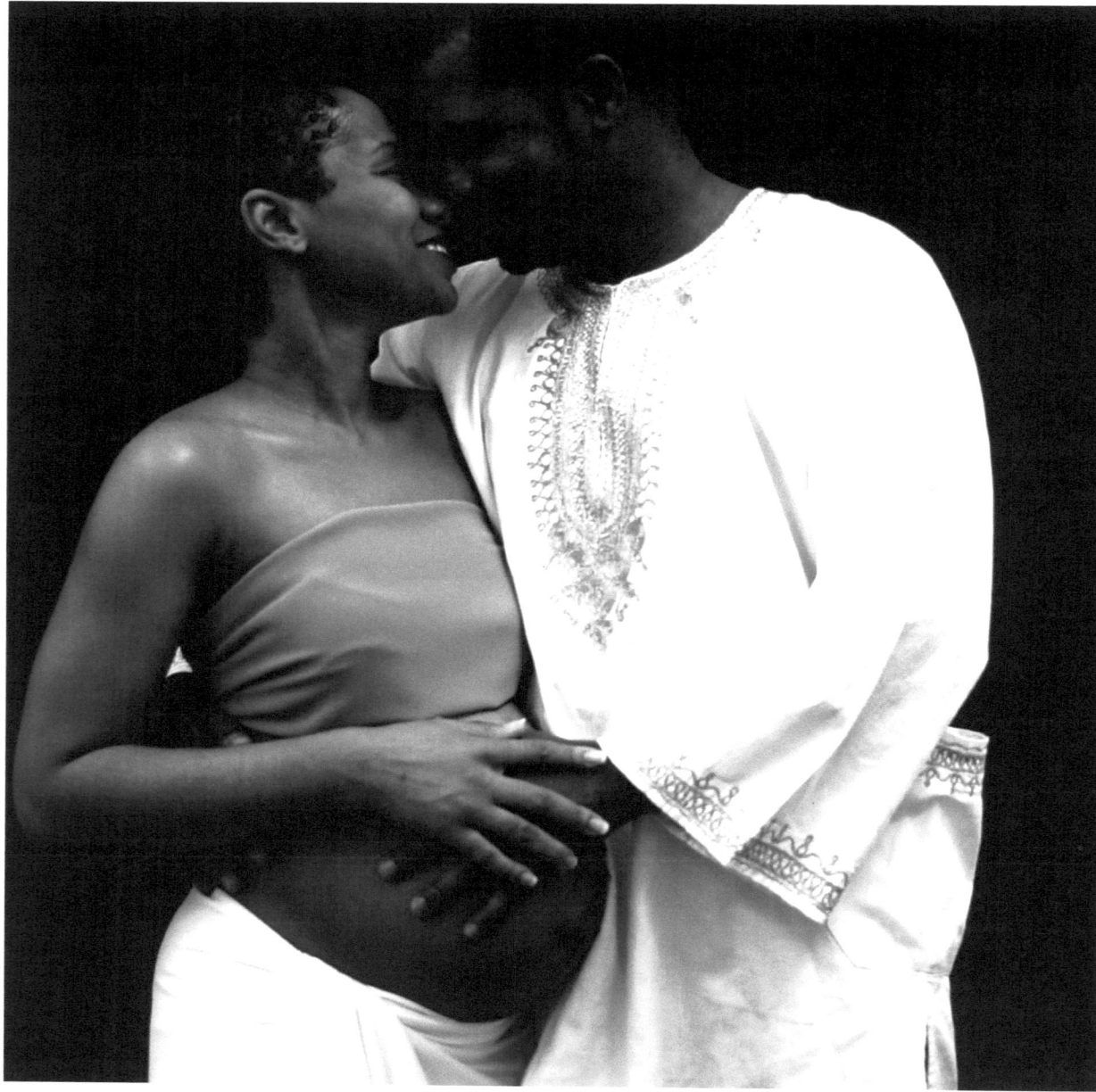

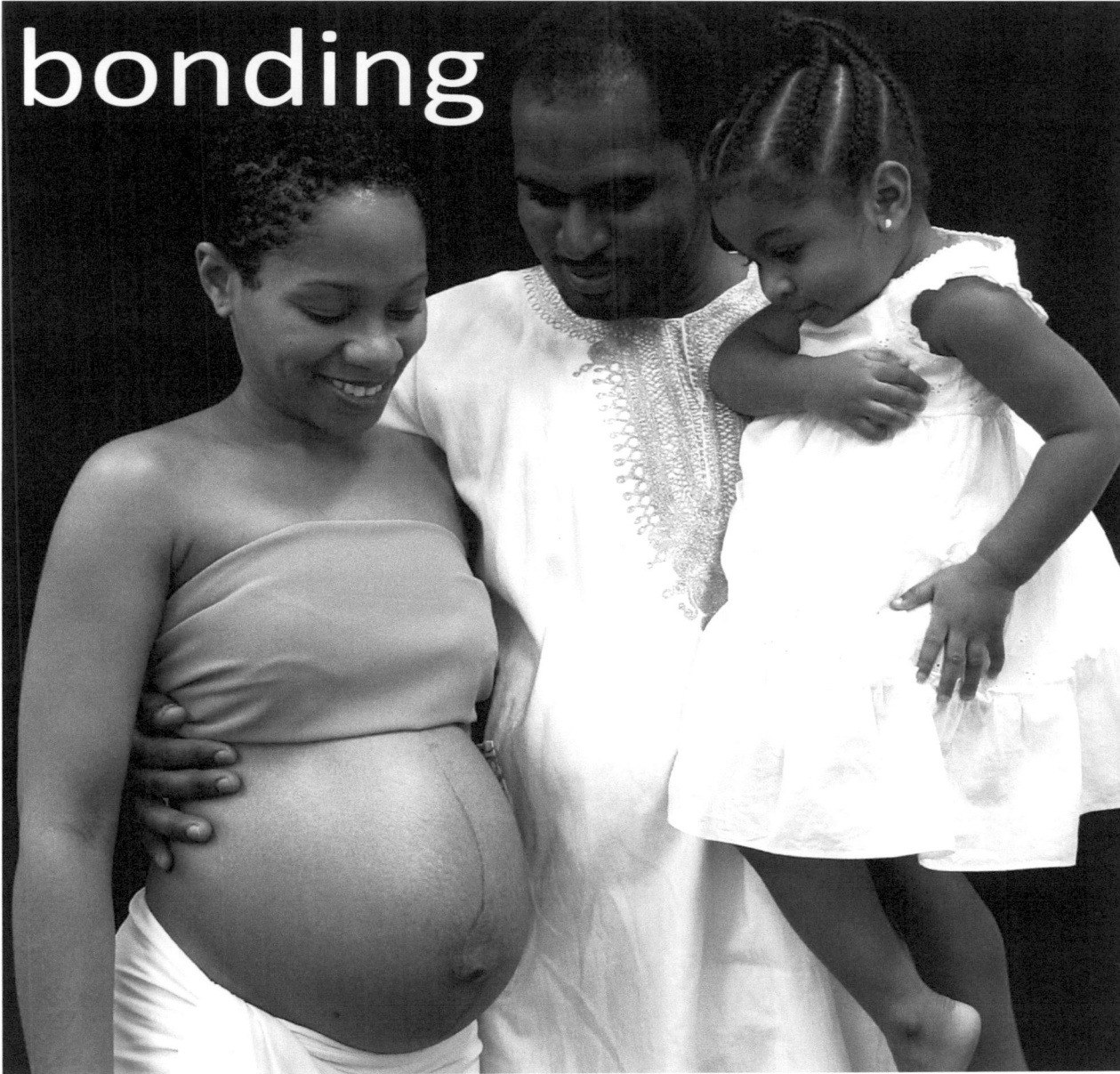

bonding

2

Labor Begins

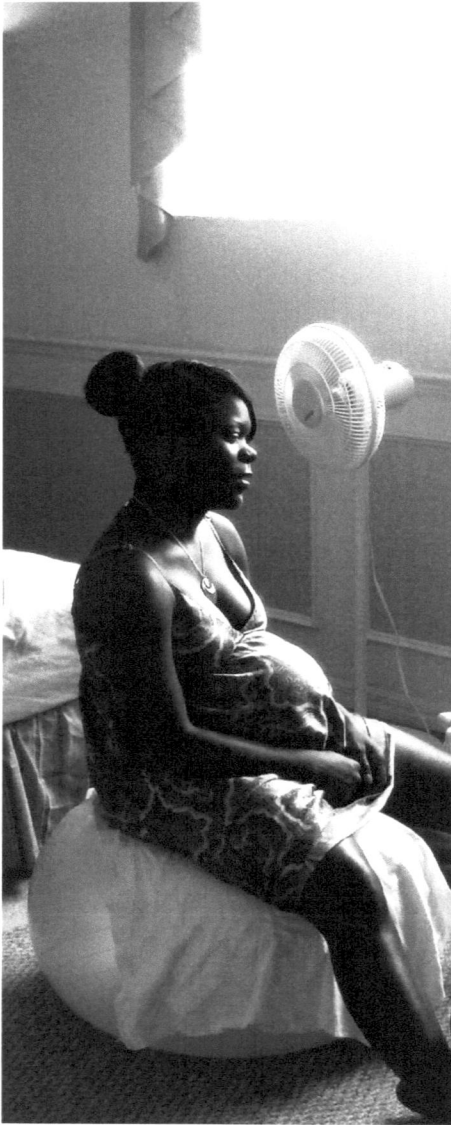

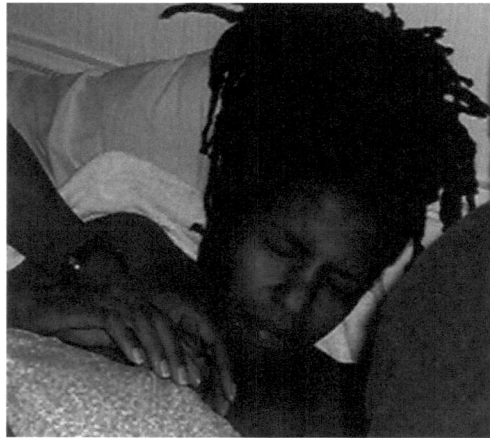

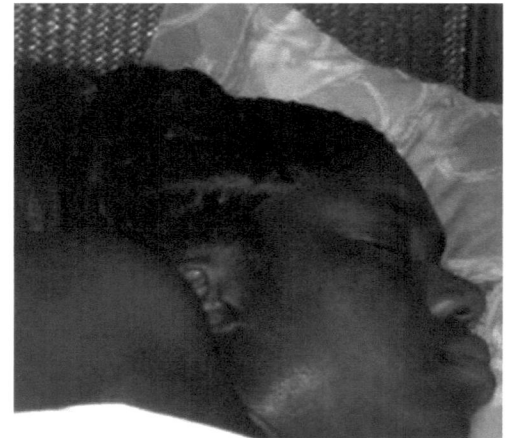

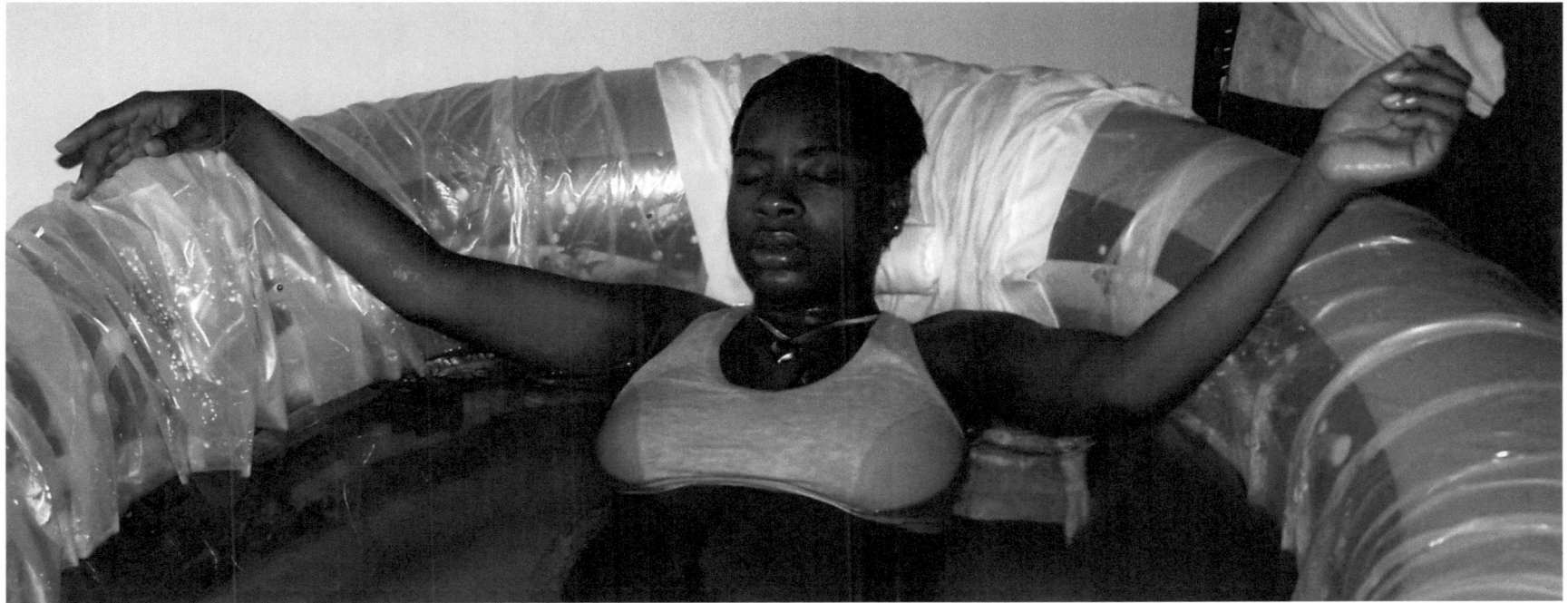

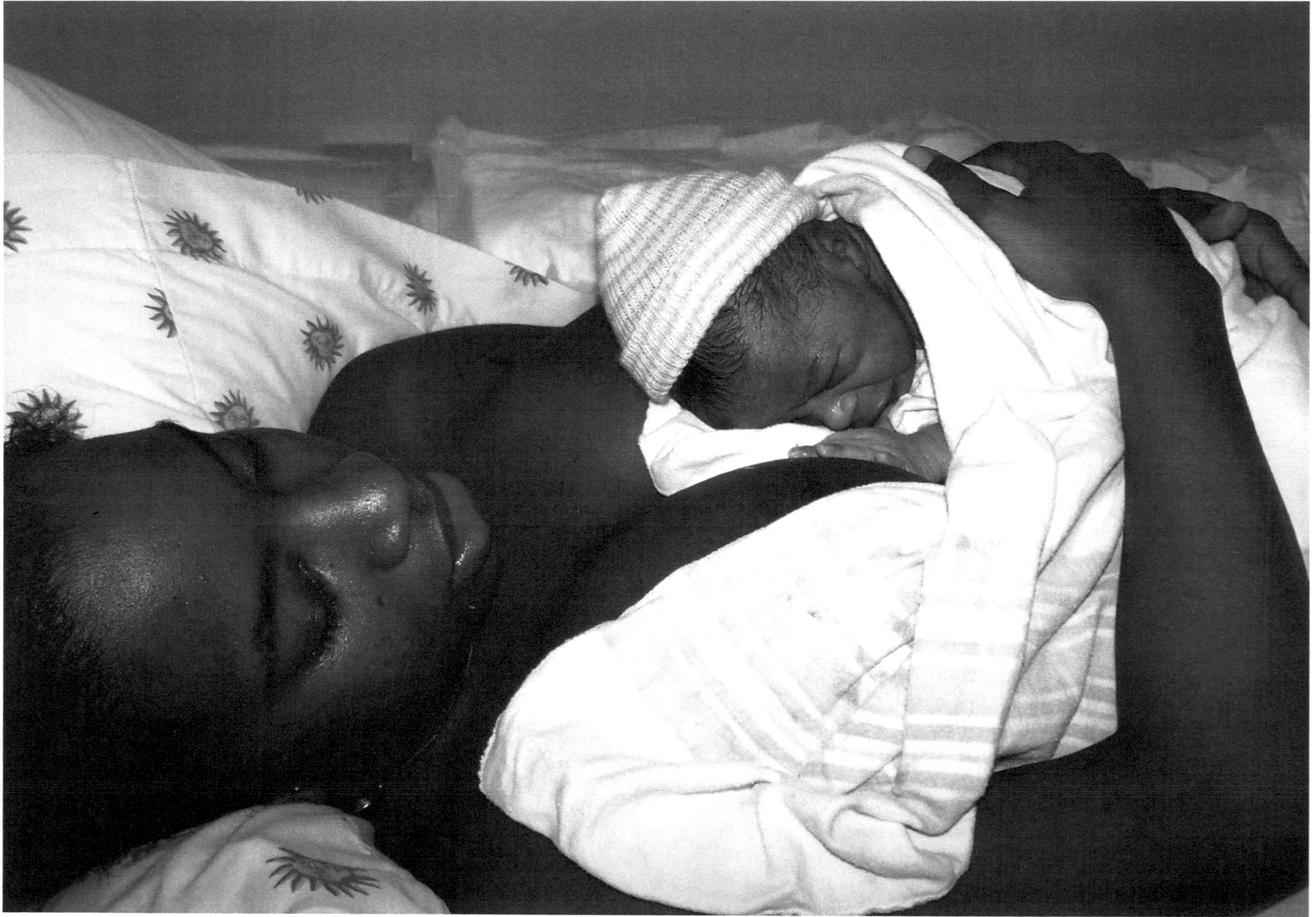

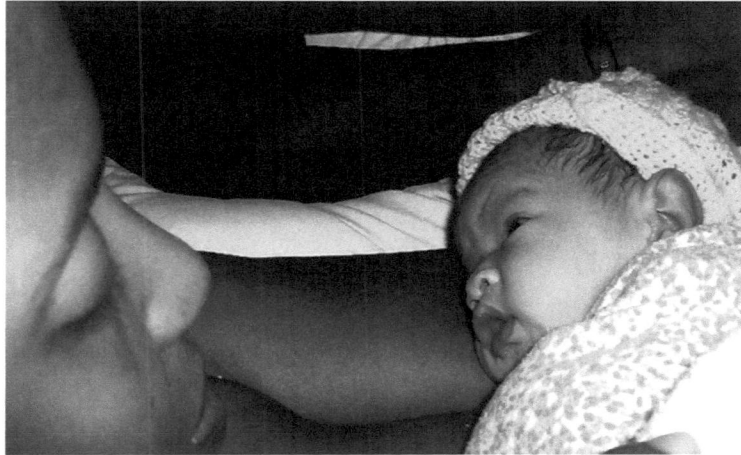

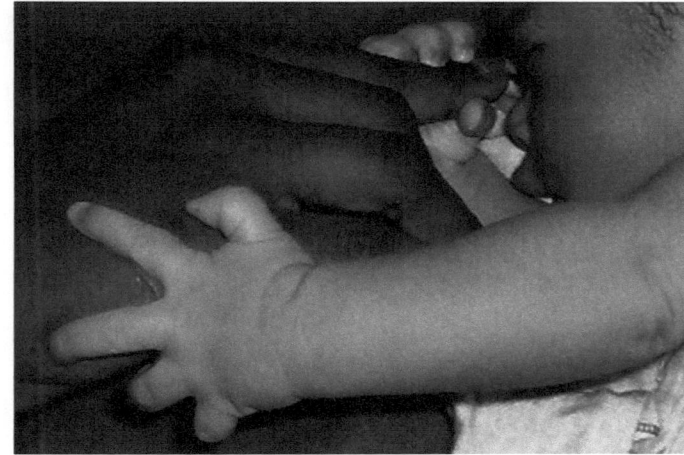

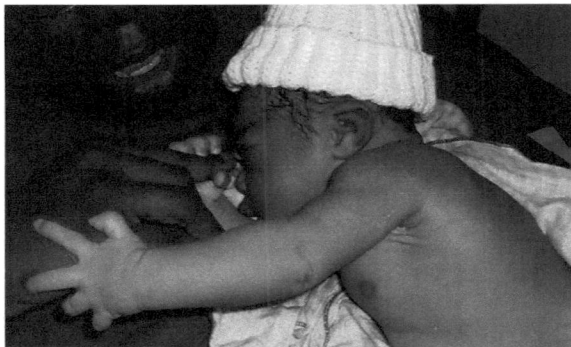

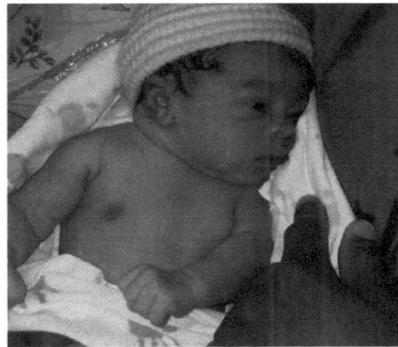

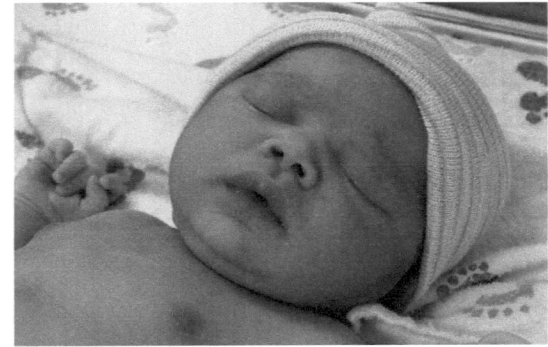

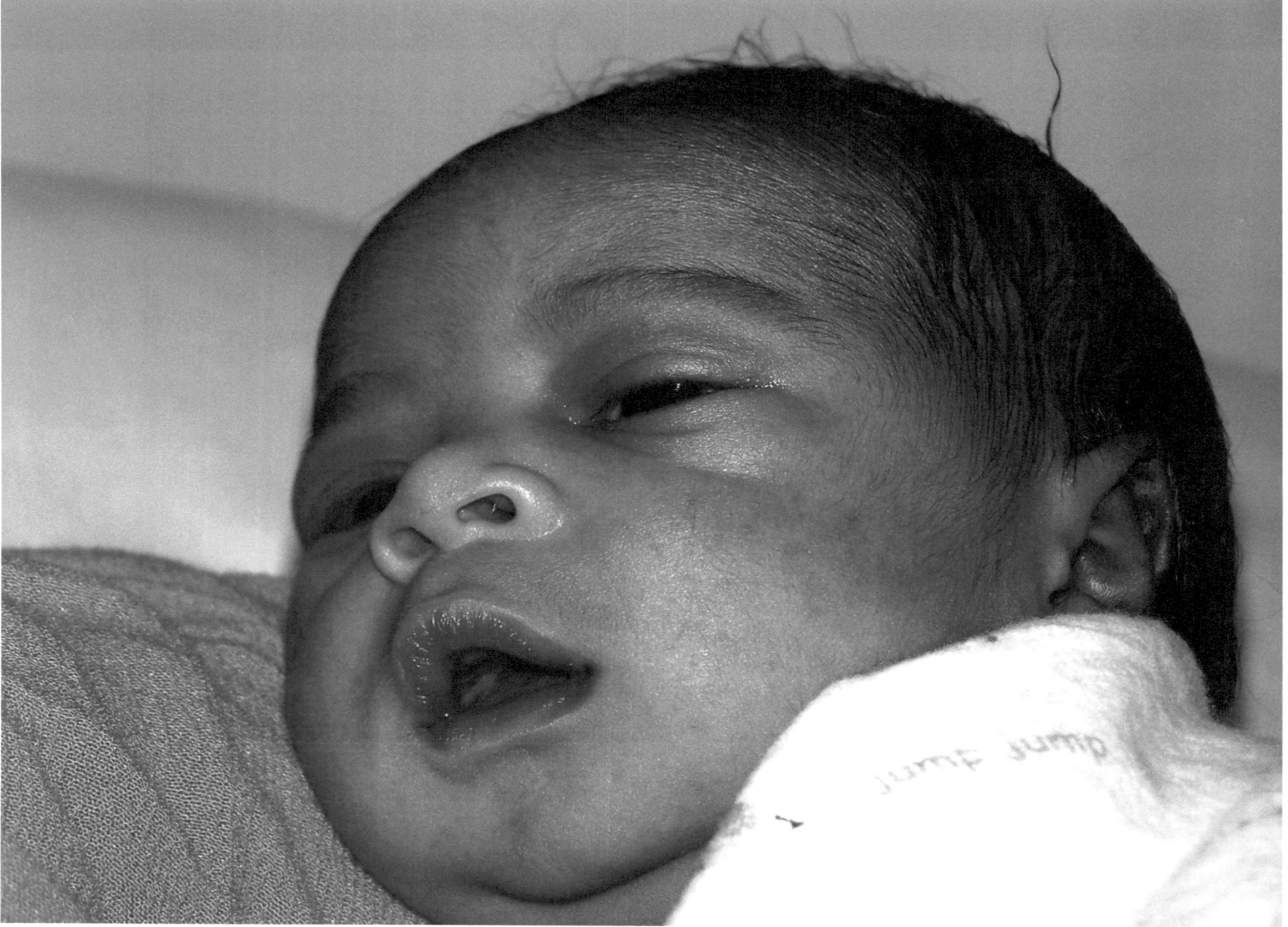

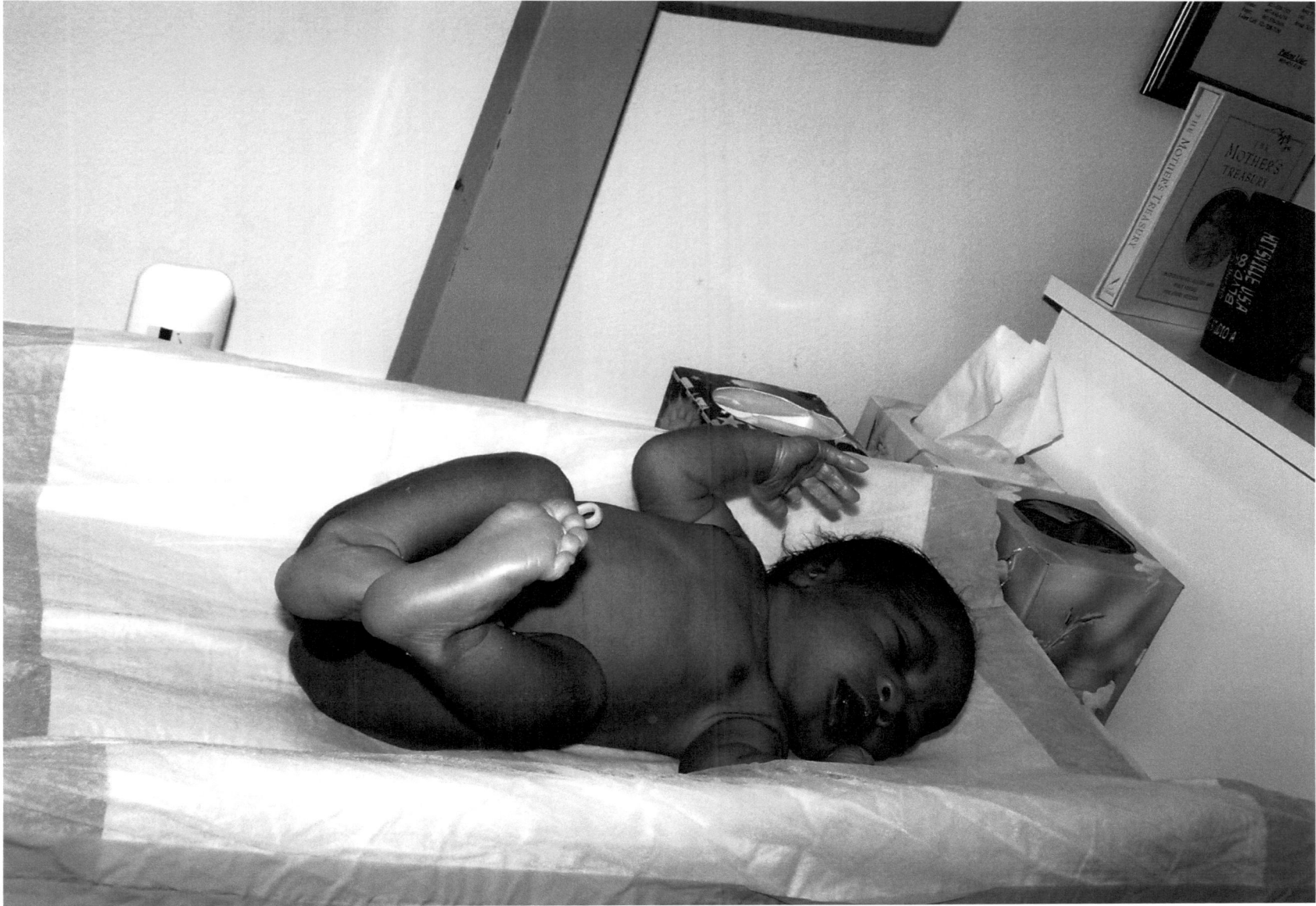

3 Family

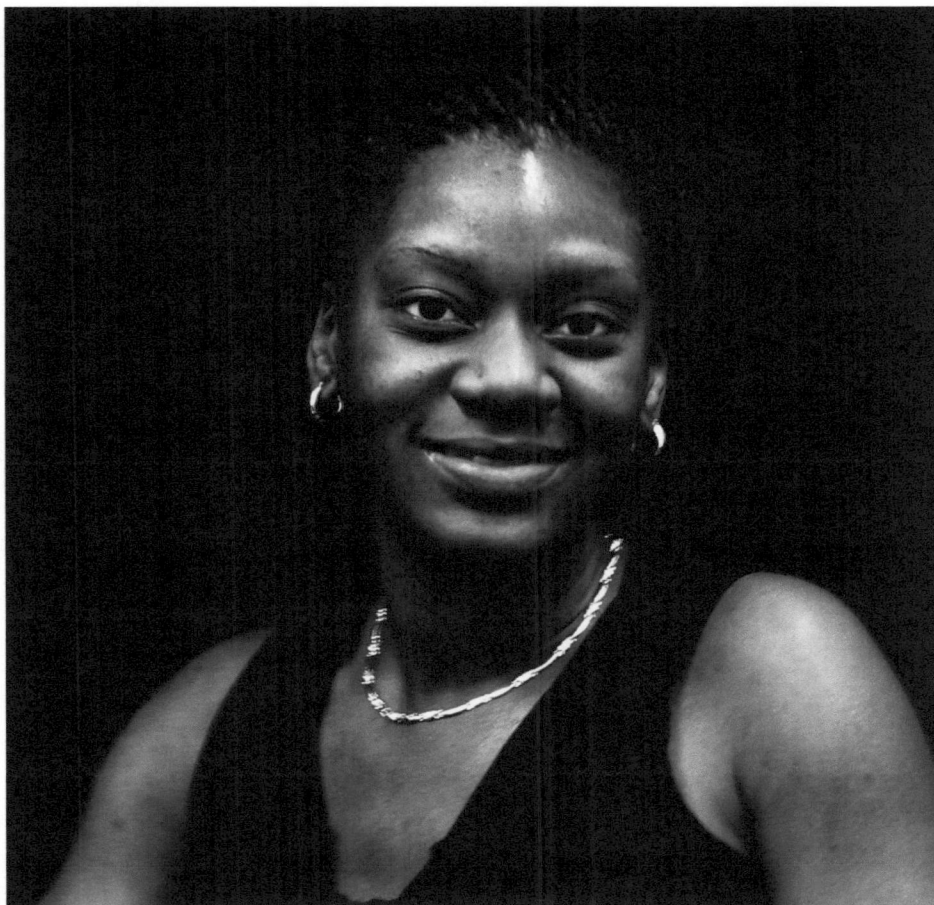

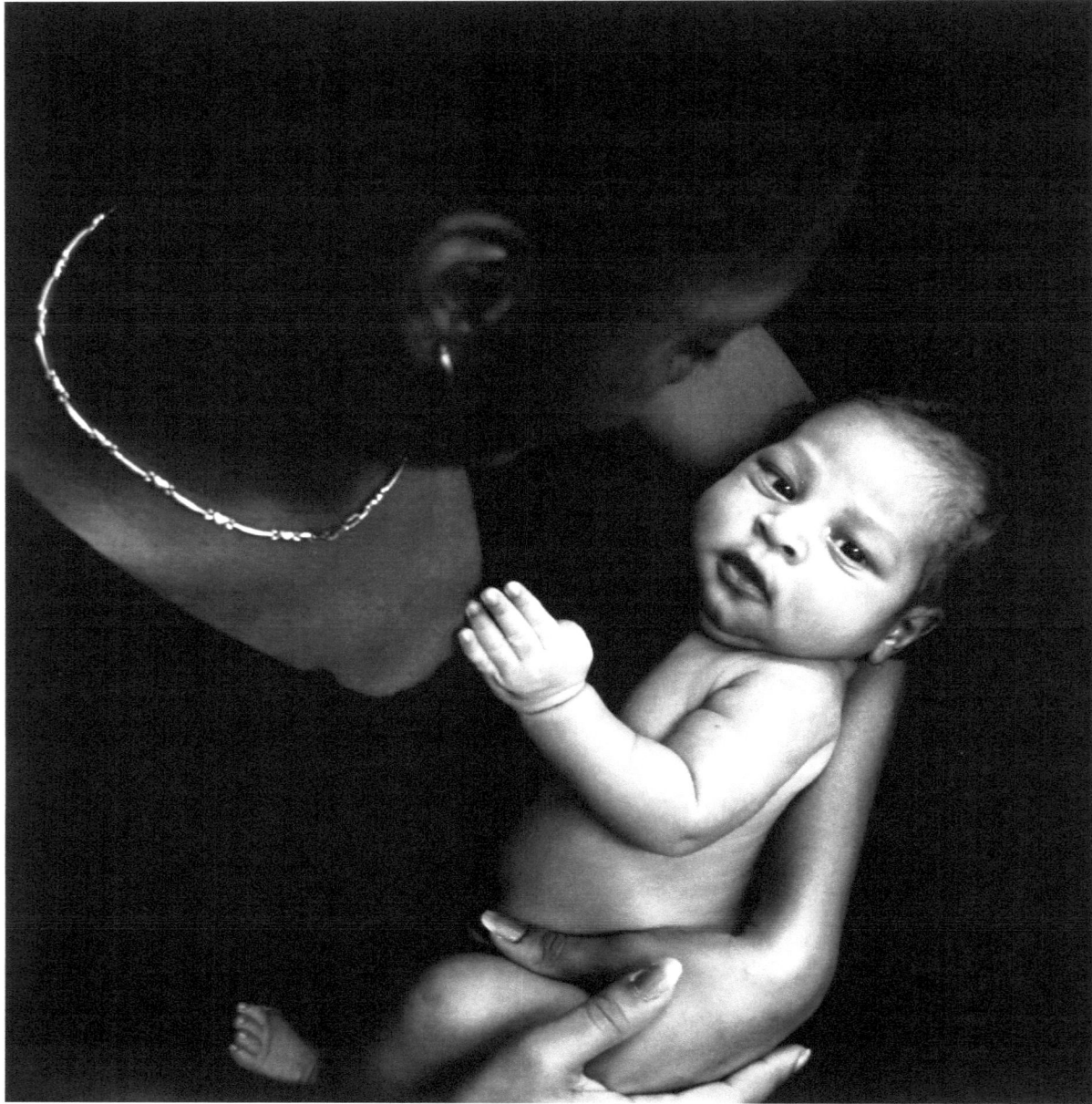

satisfaction

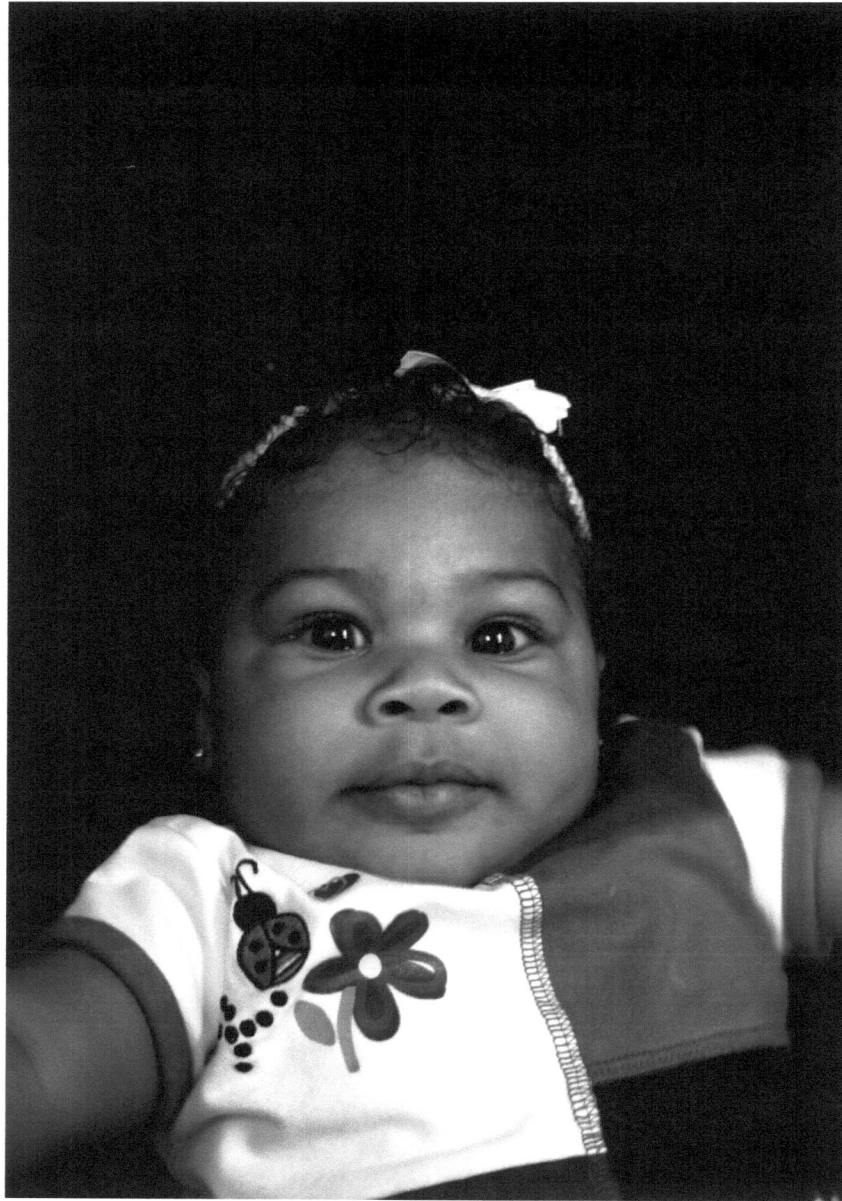

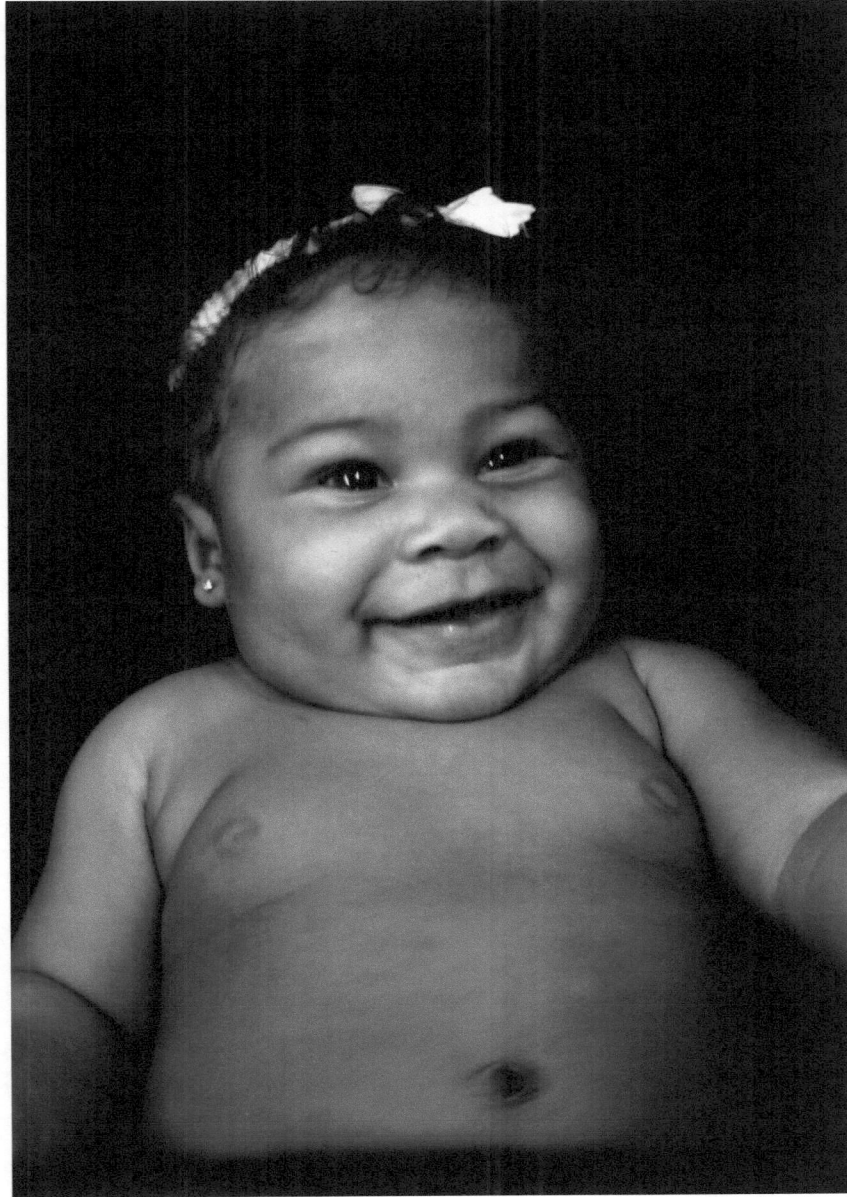

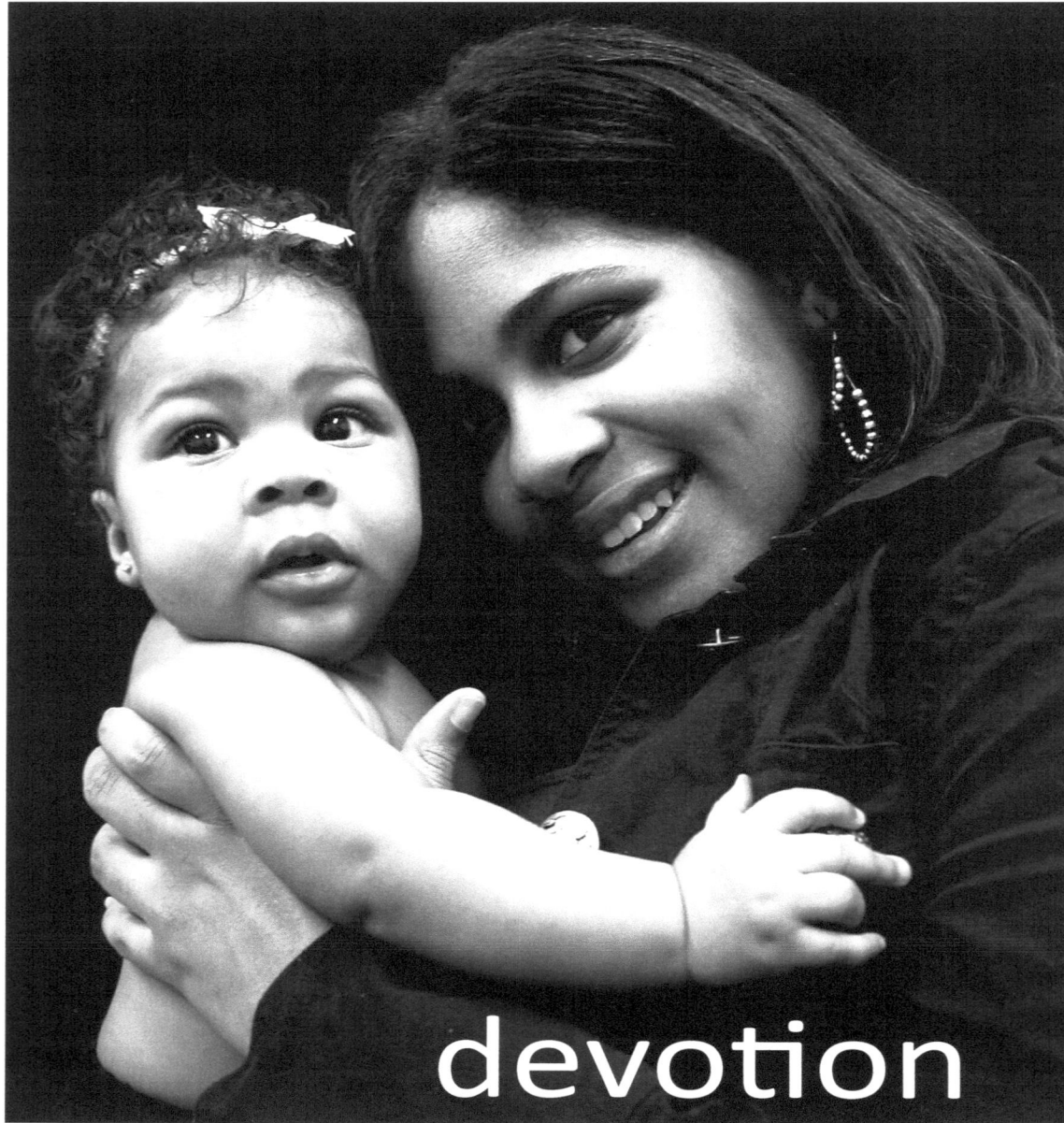

devotion

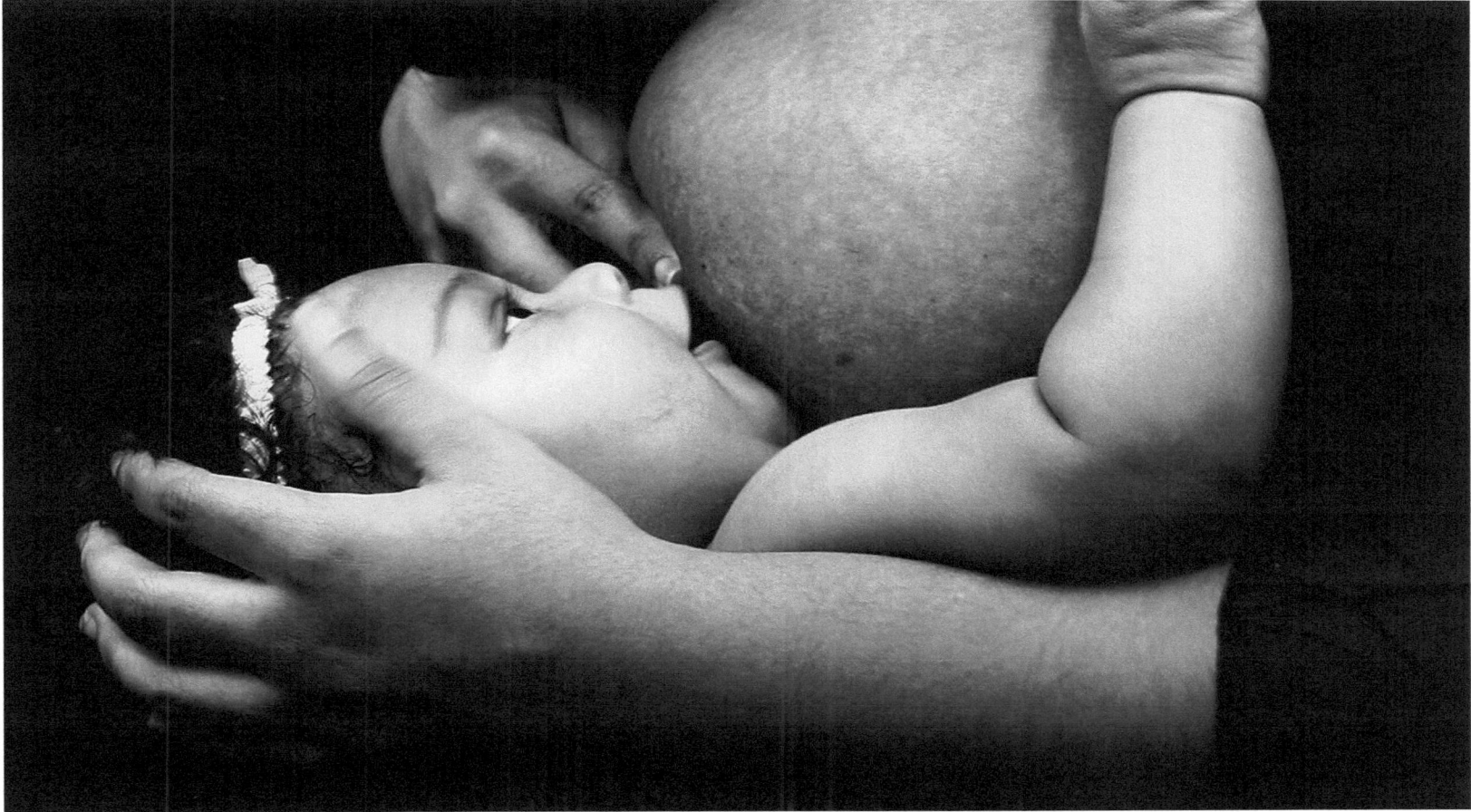

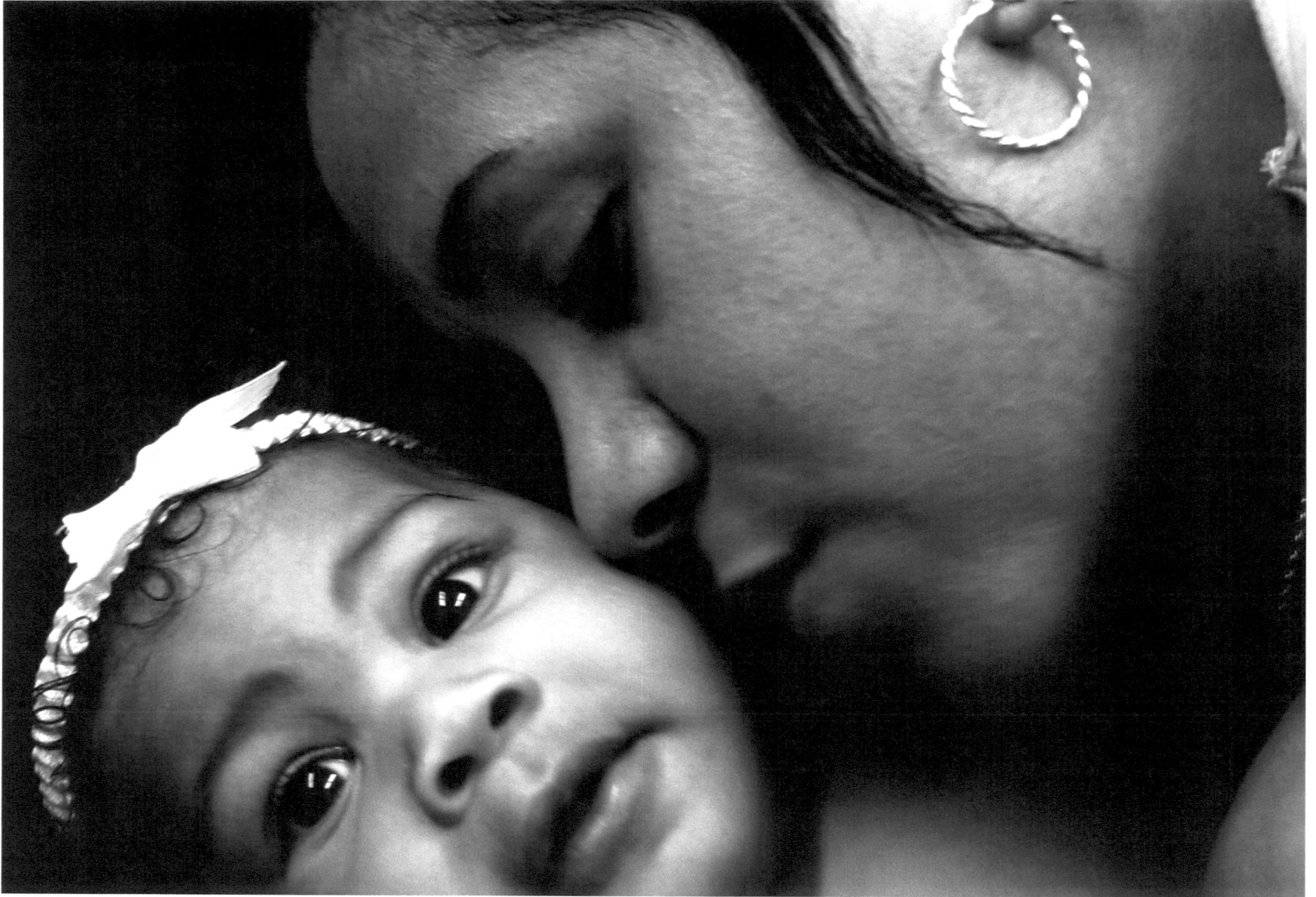

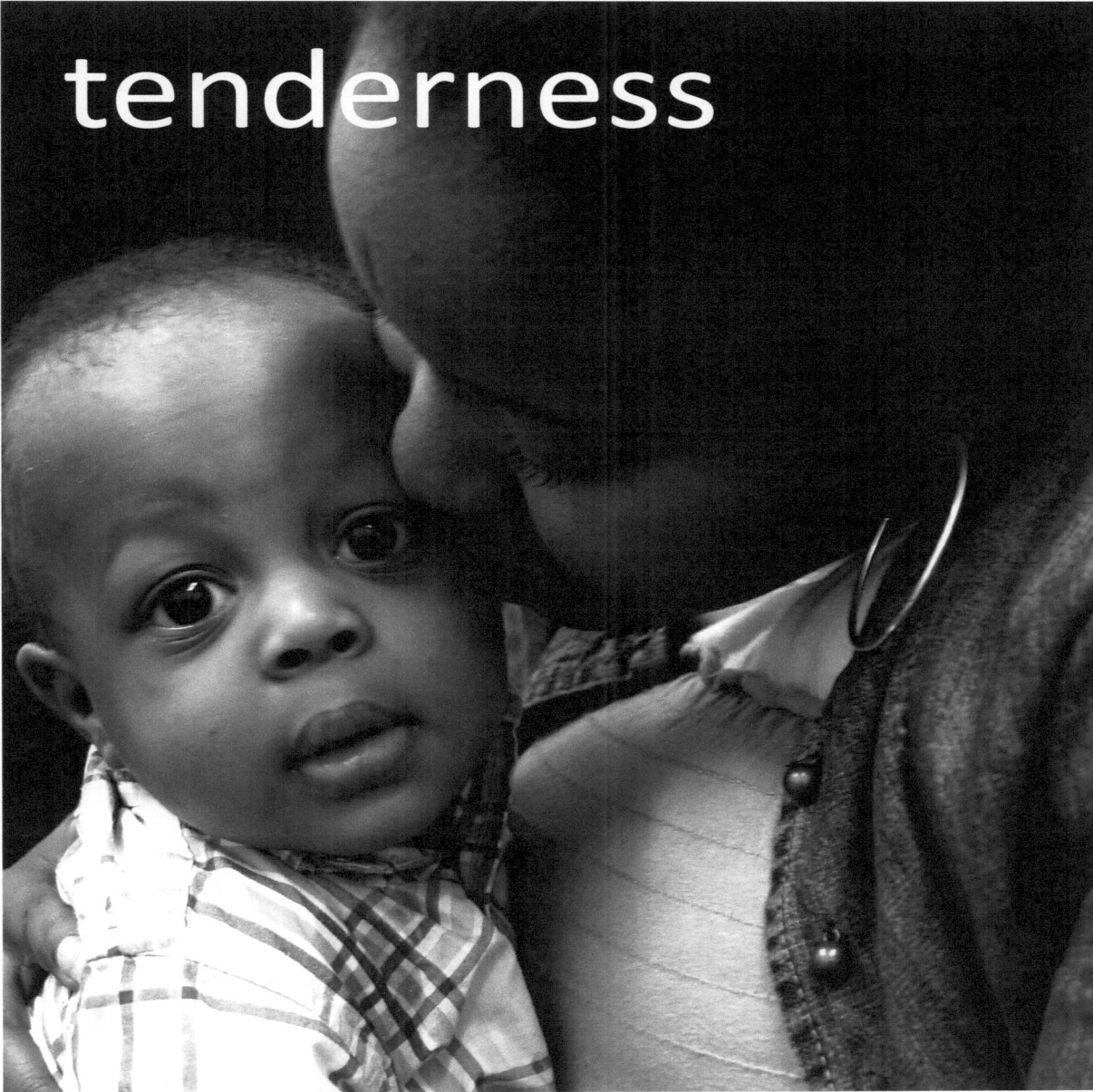

tenderness

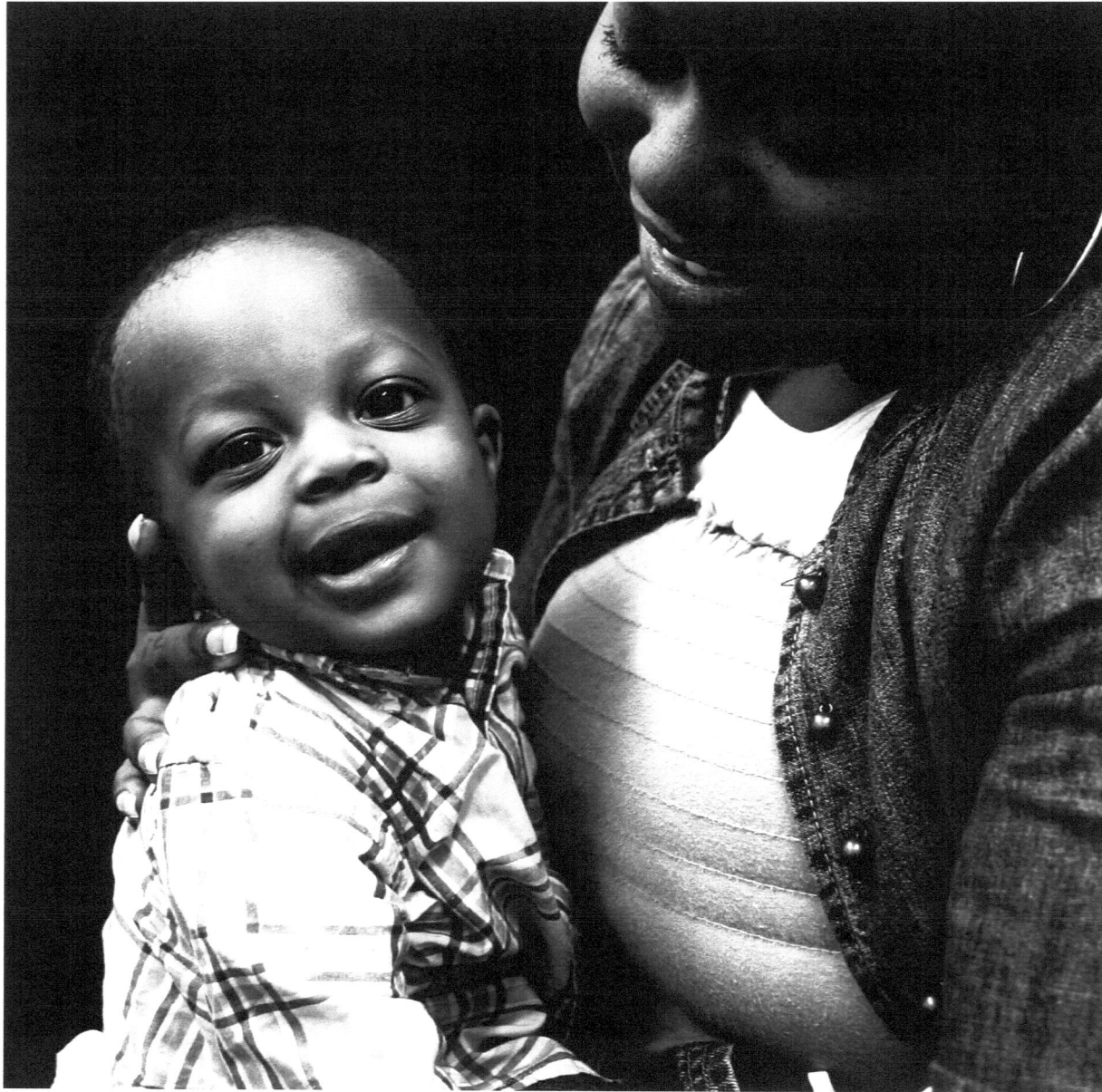

hope

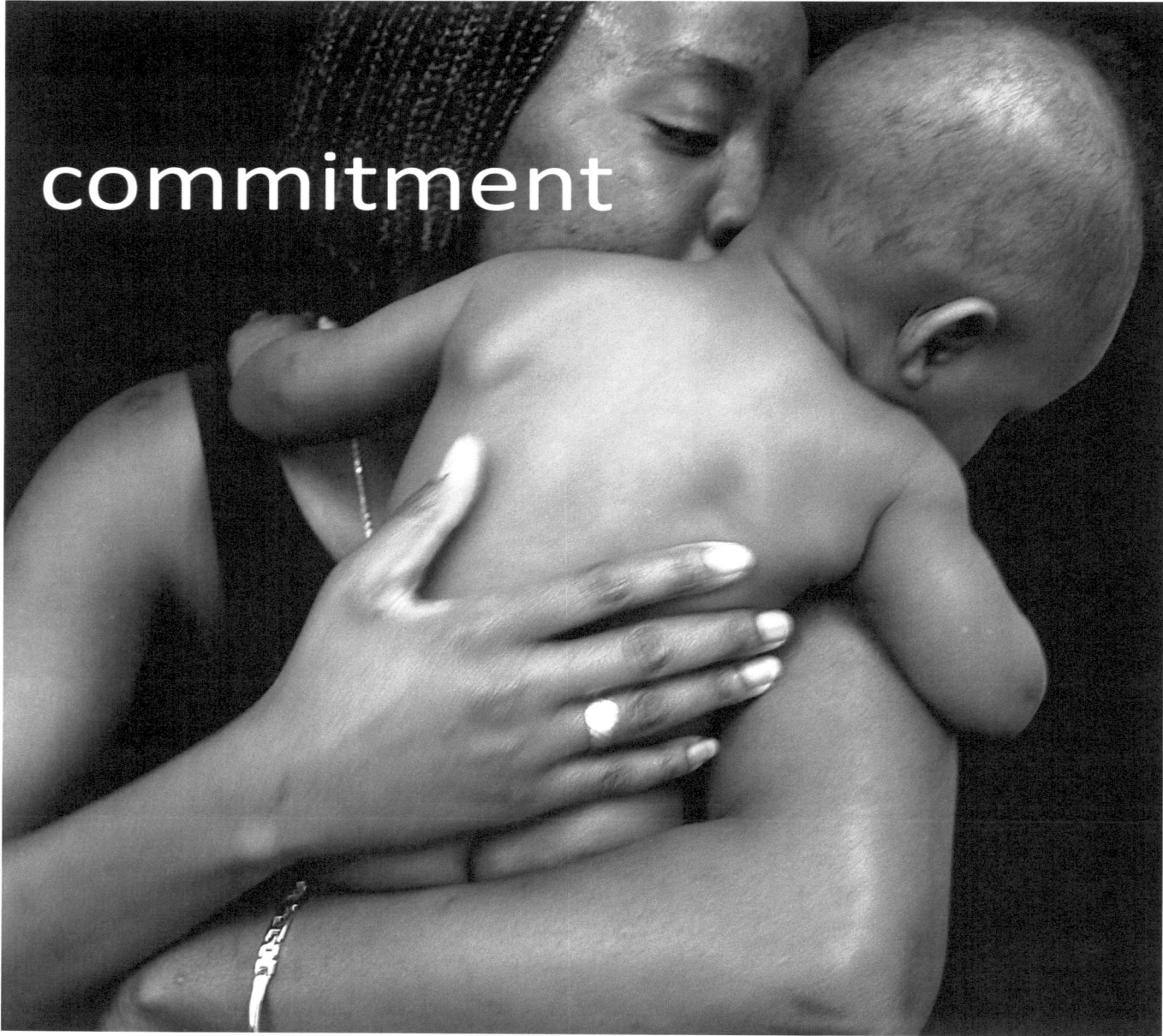

commitment

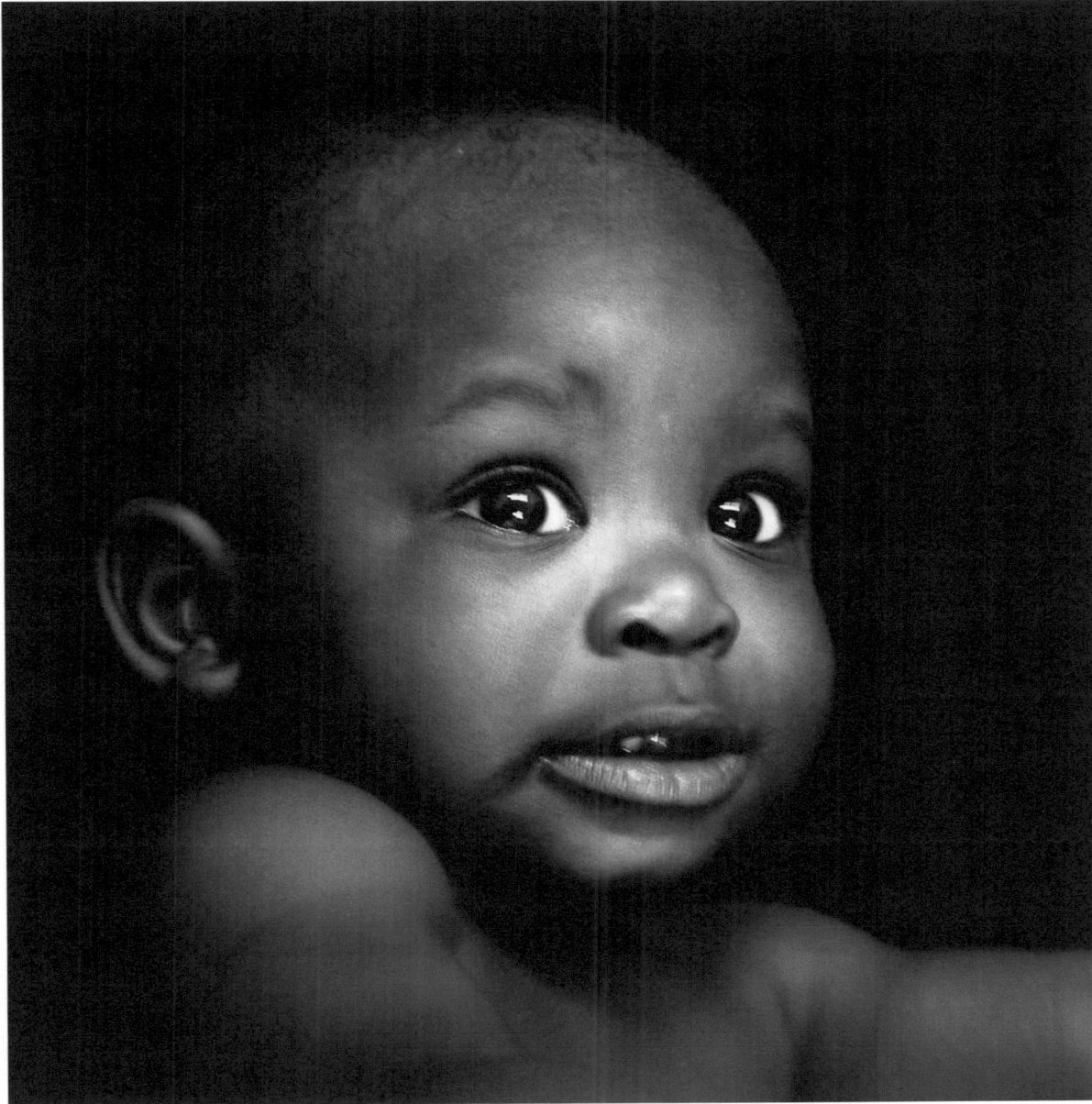

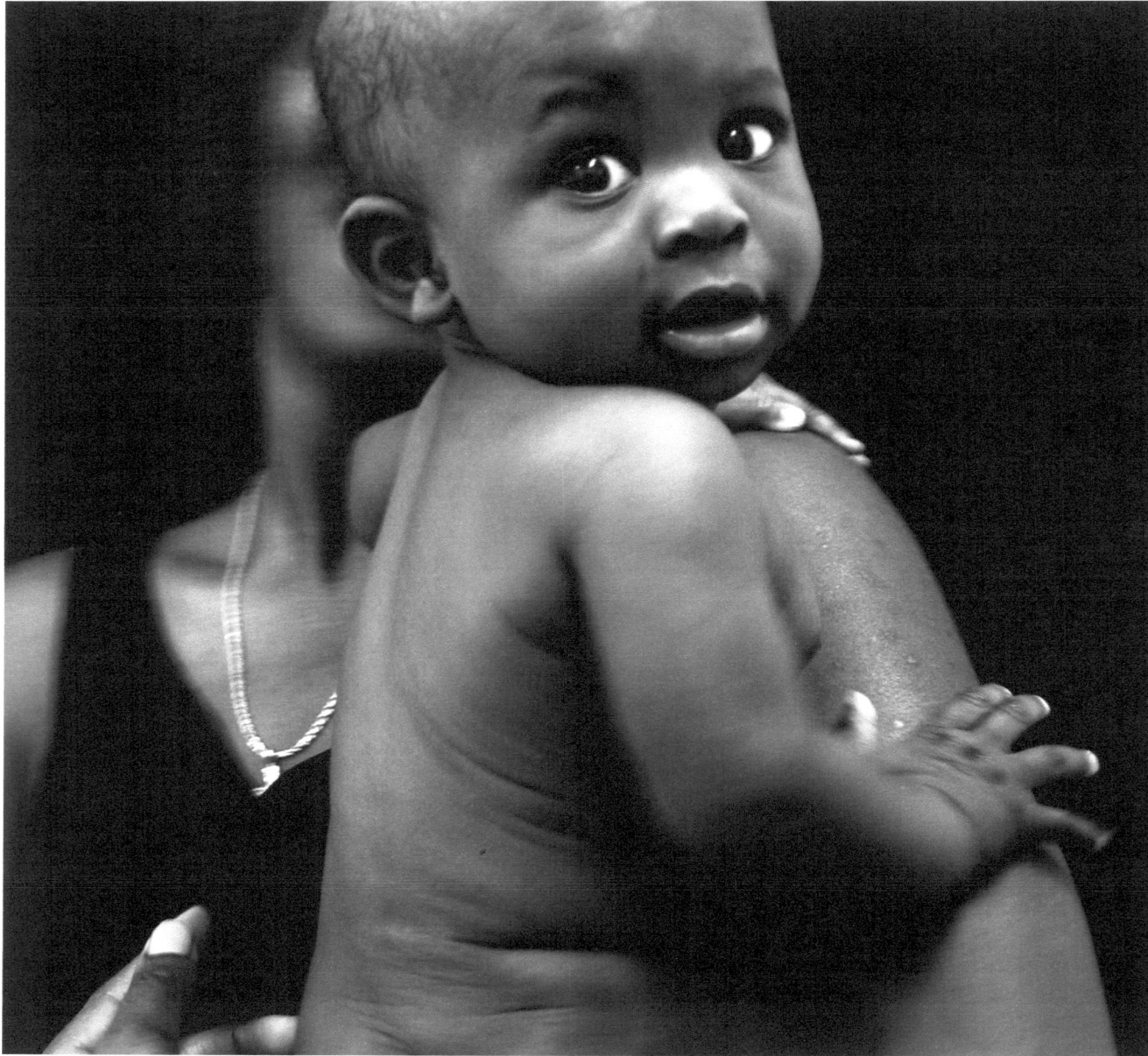

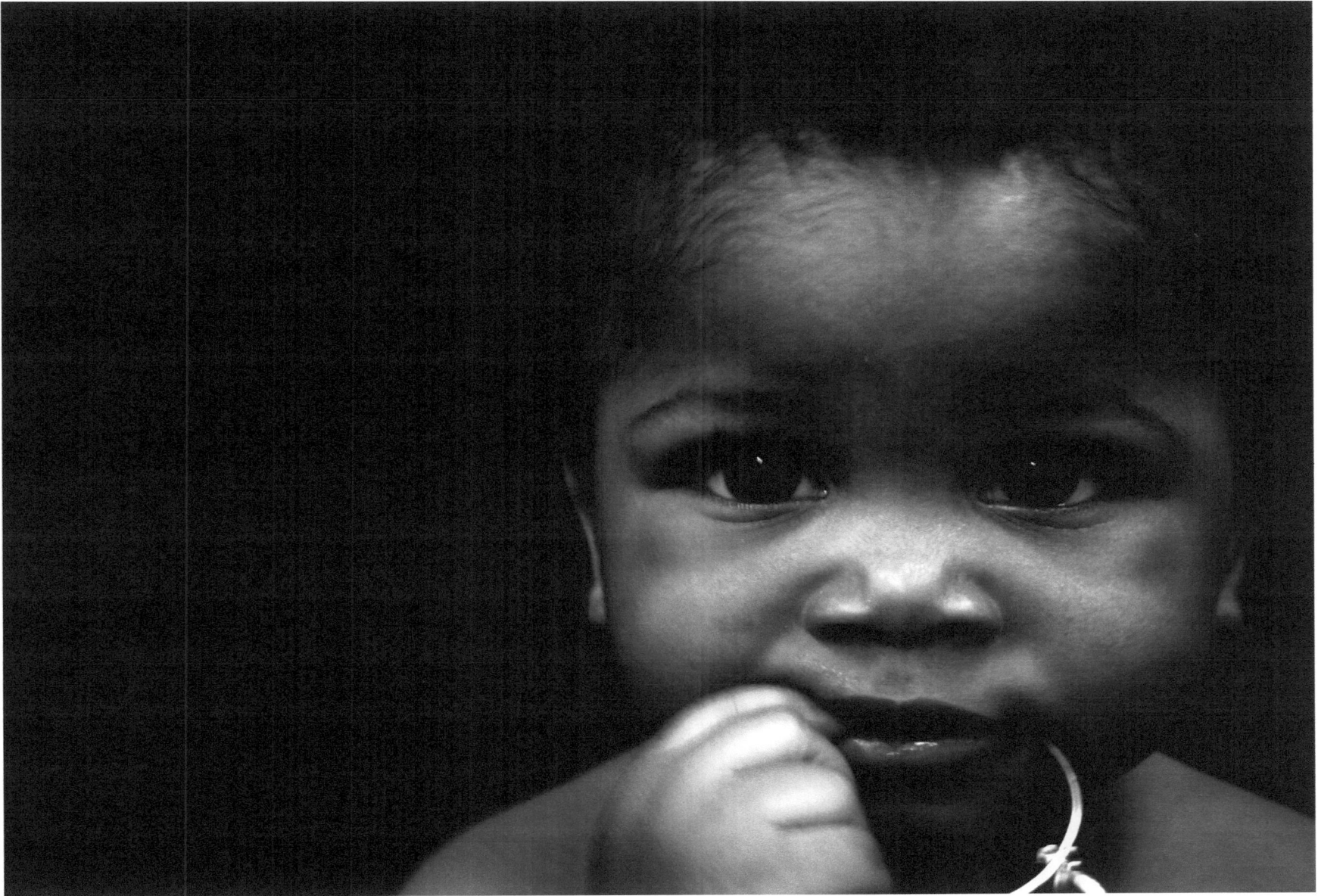

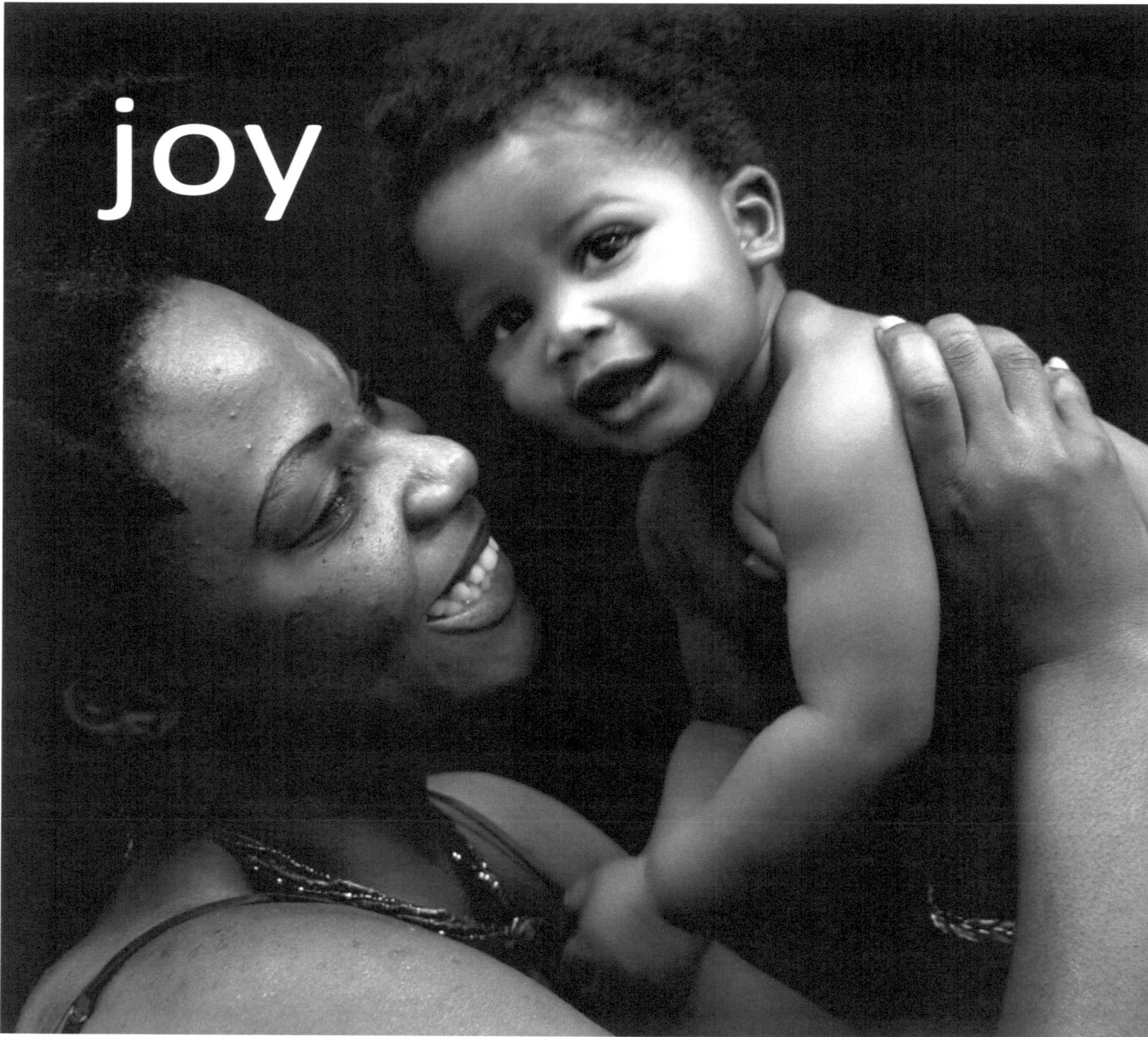

joy

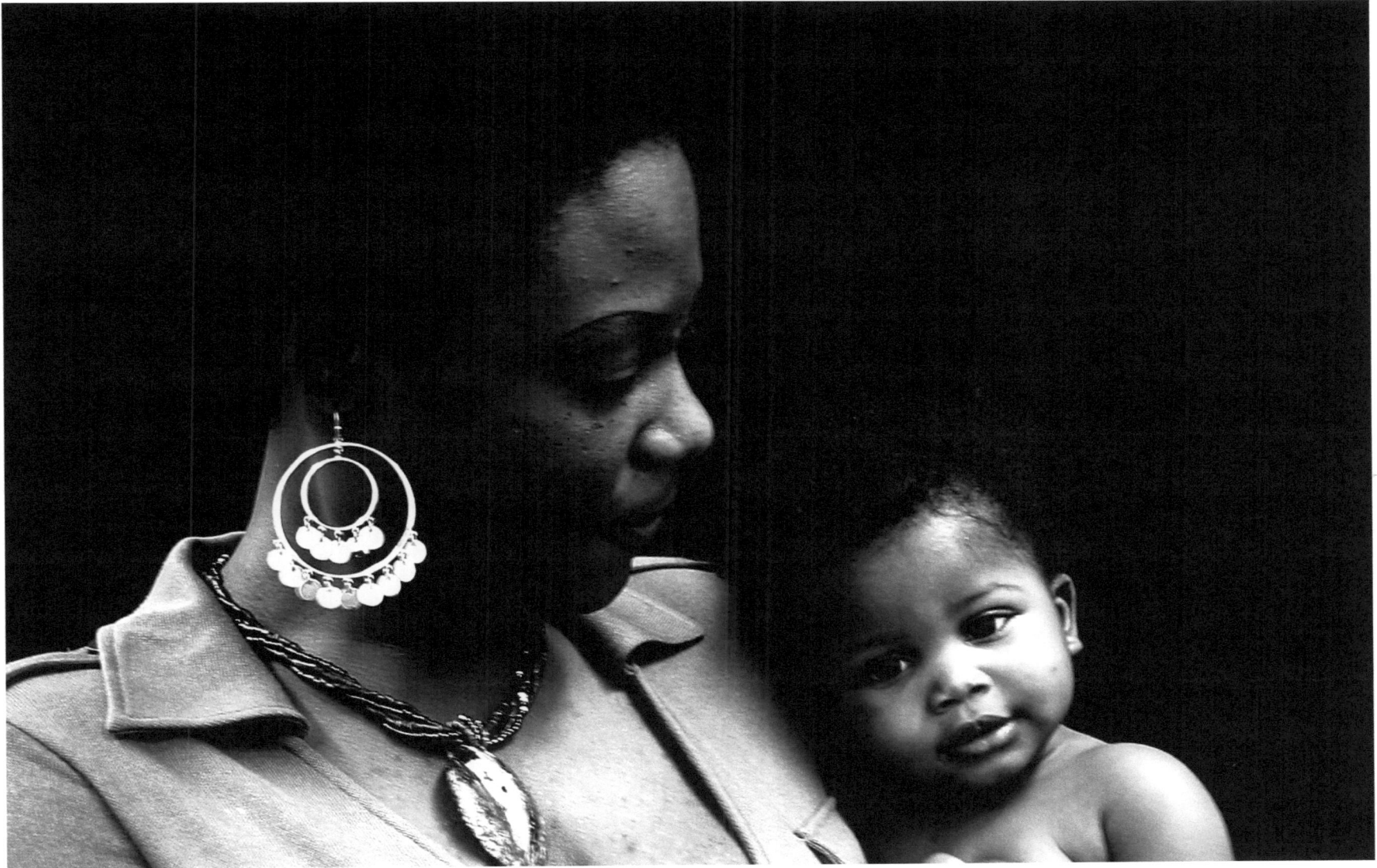

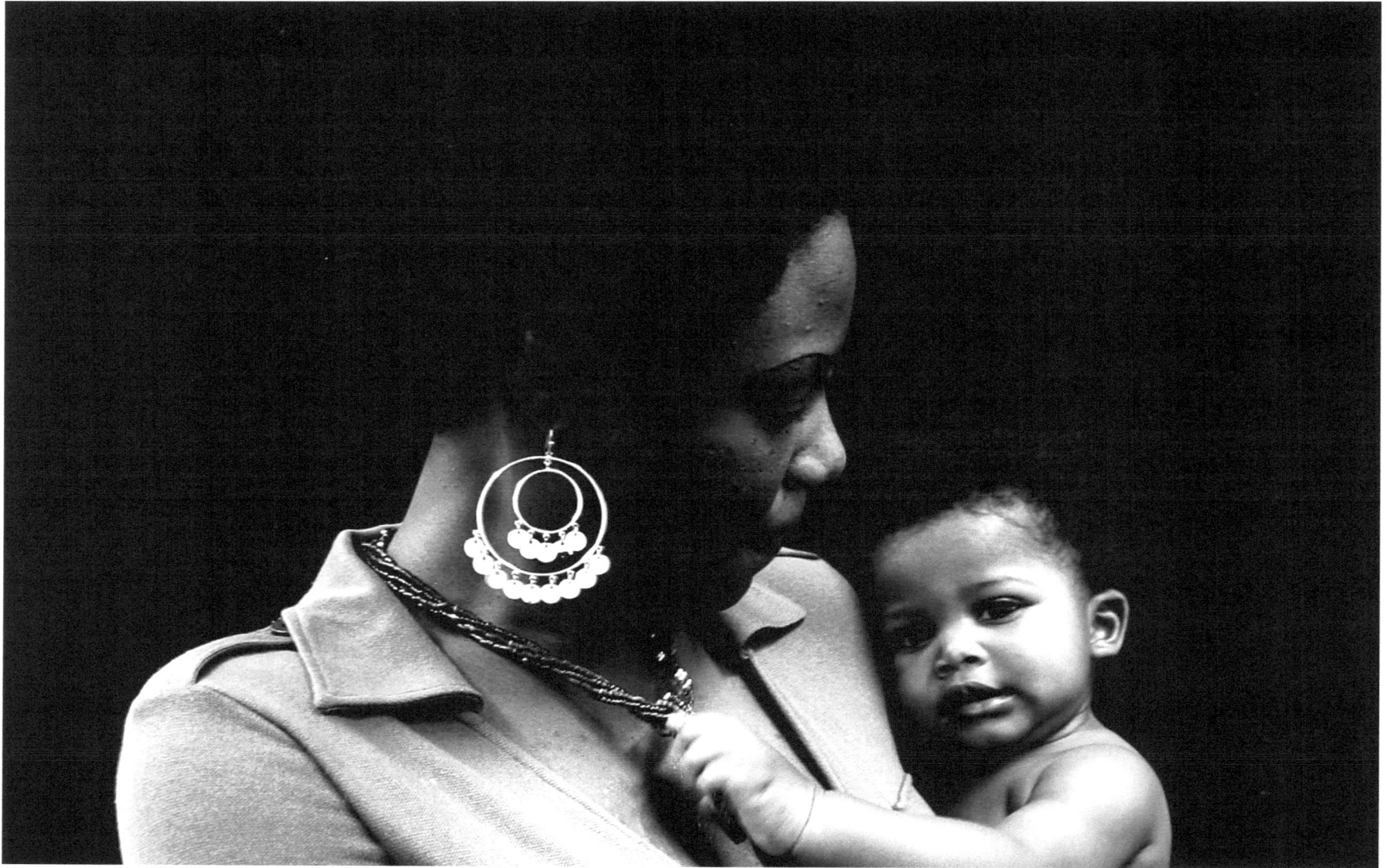

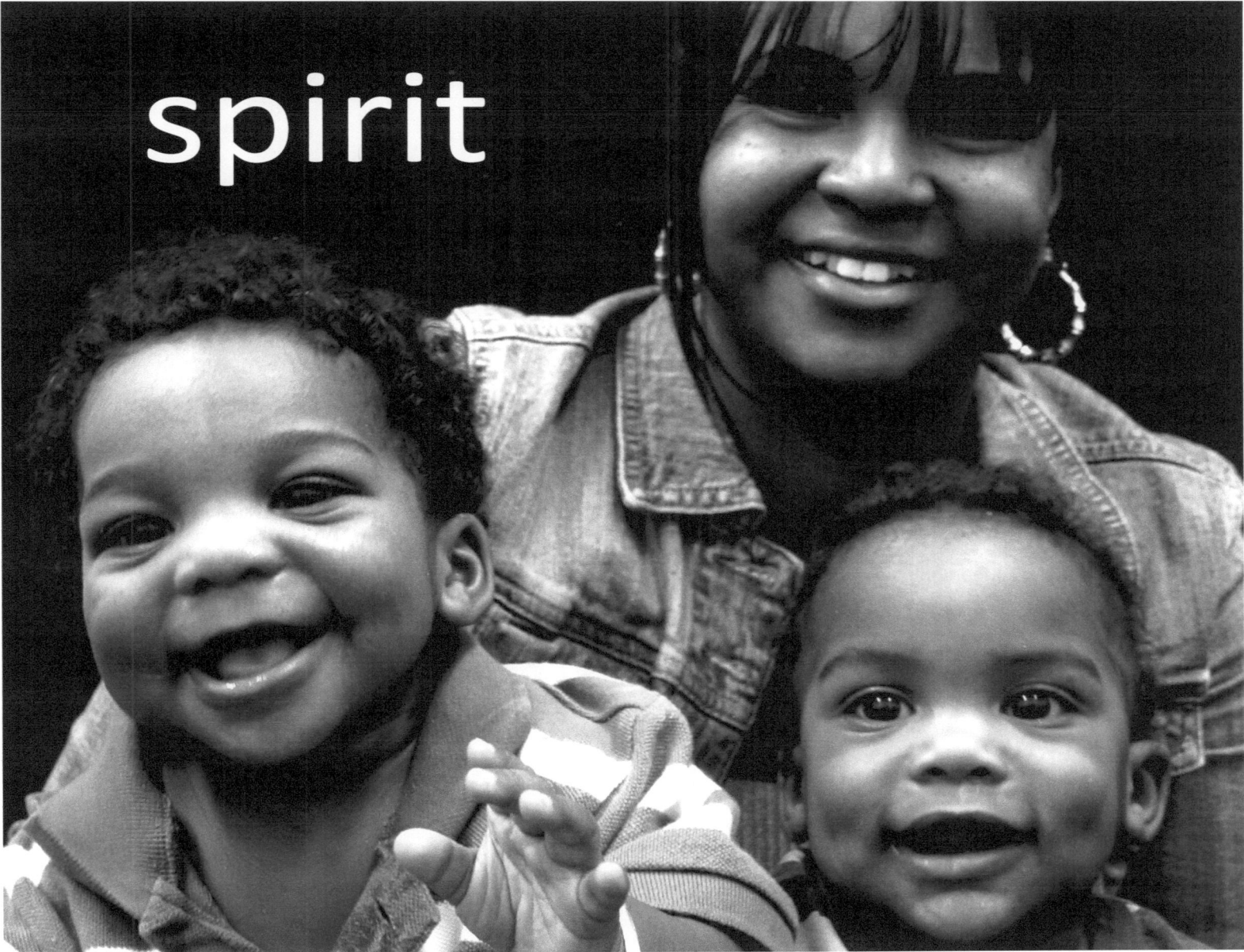

spirit

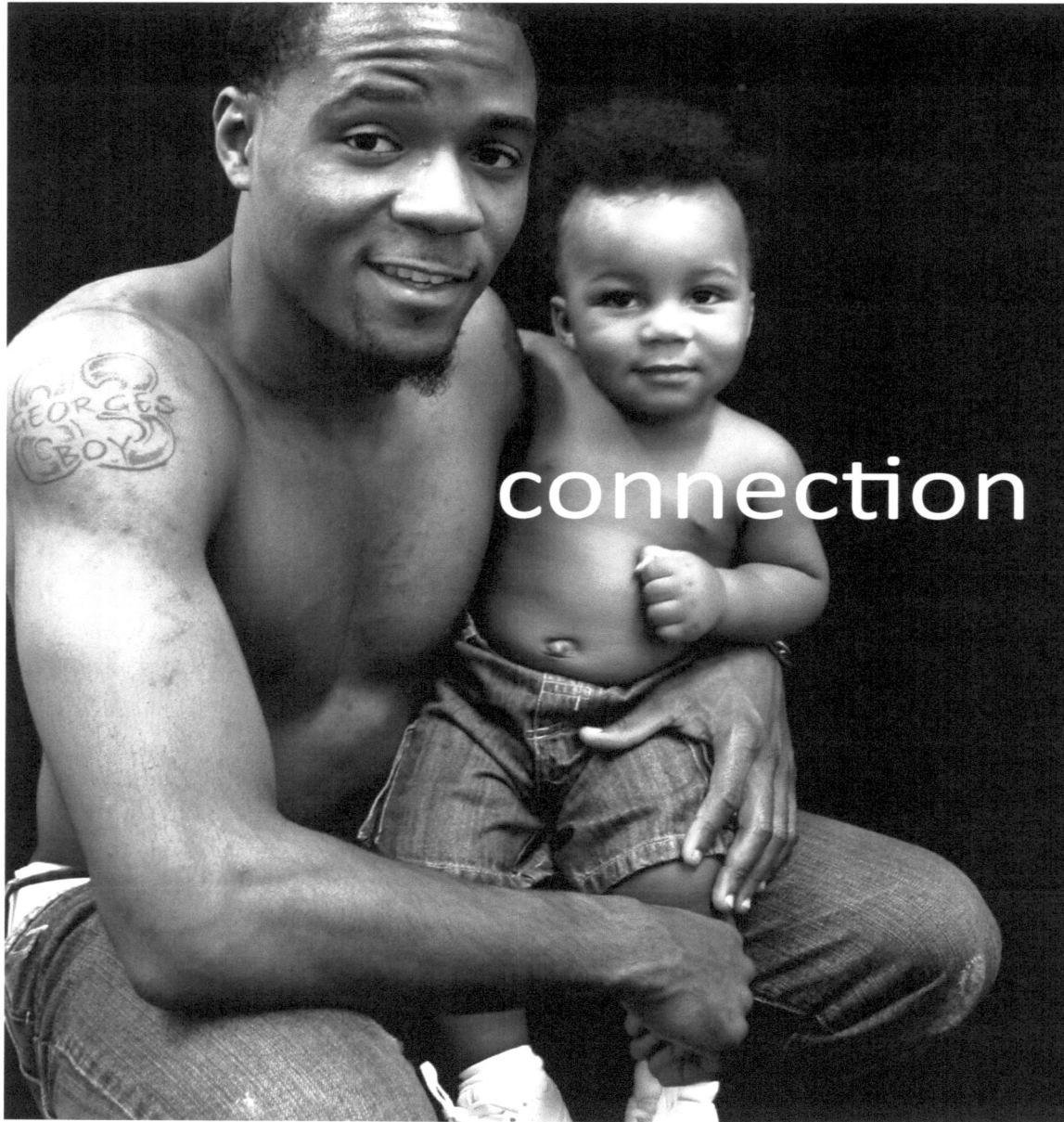

connection

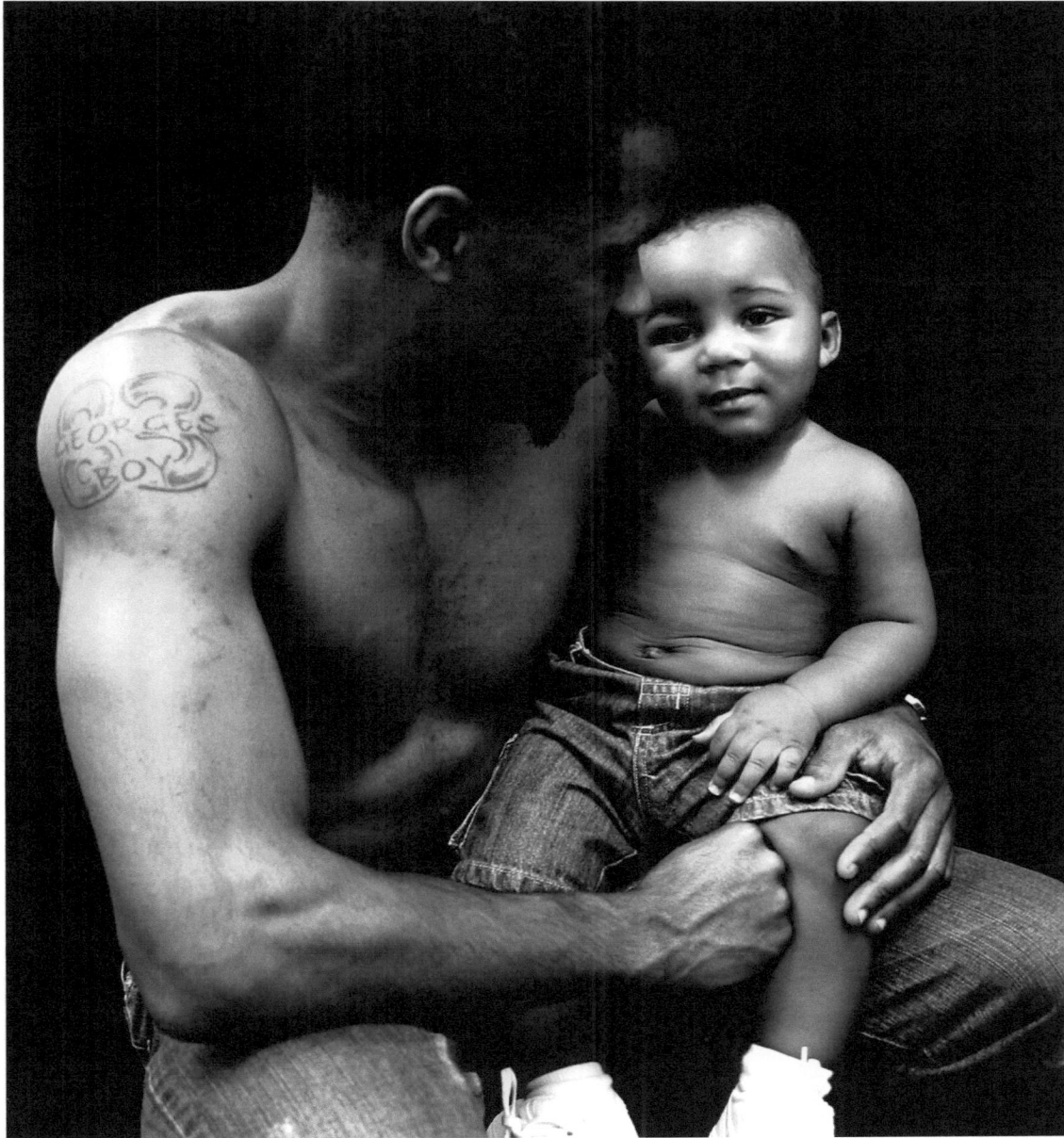

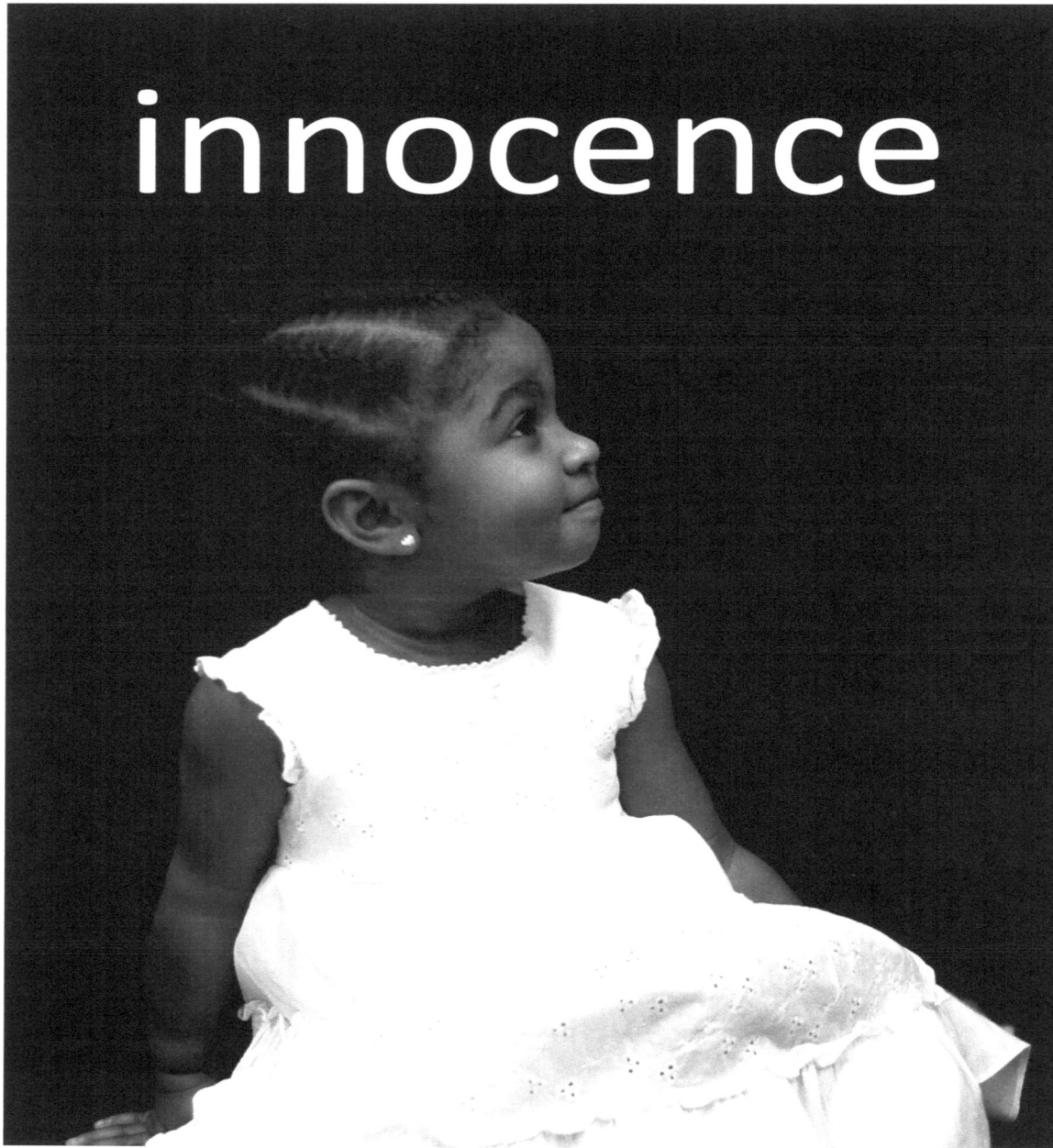

innocence

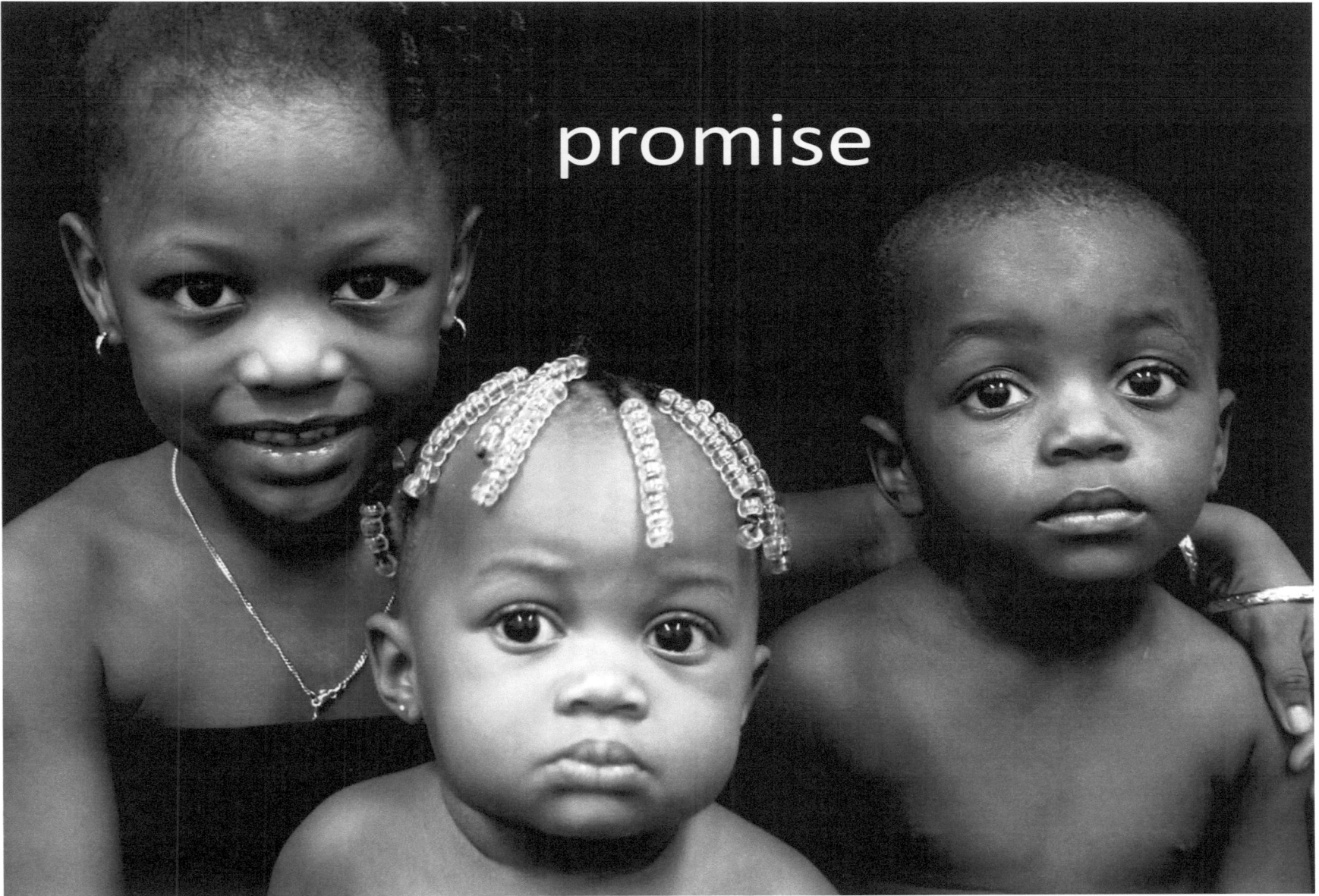

promise

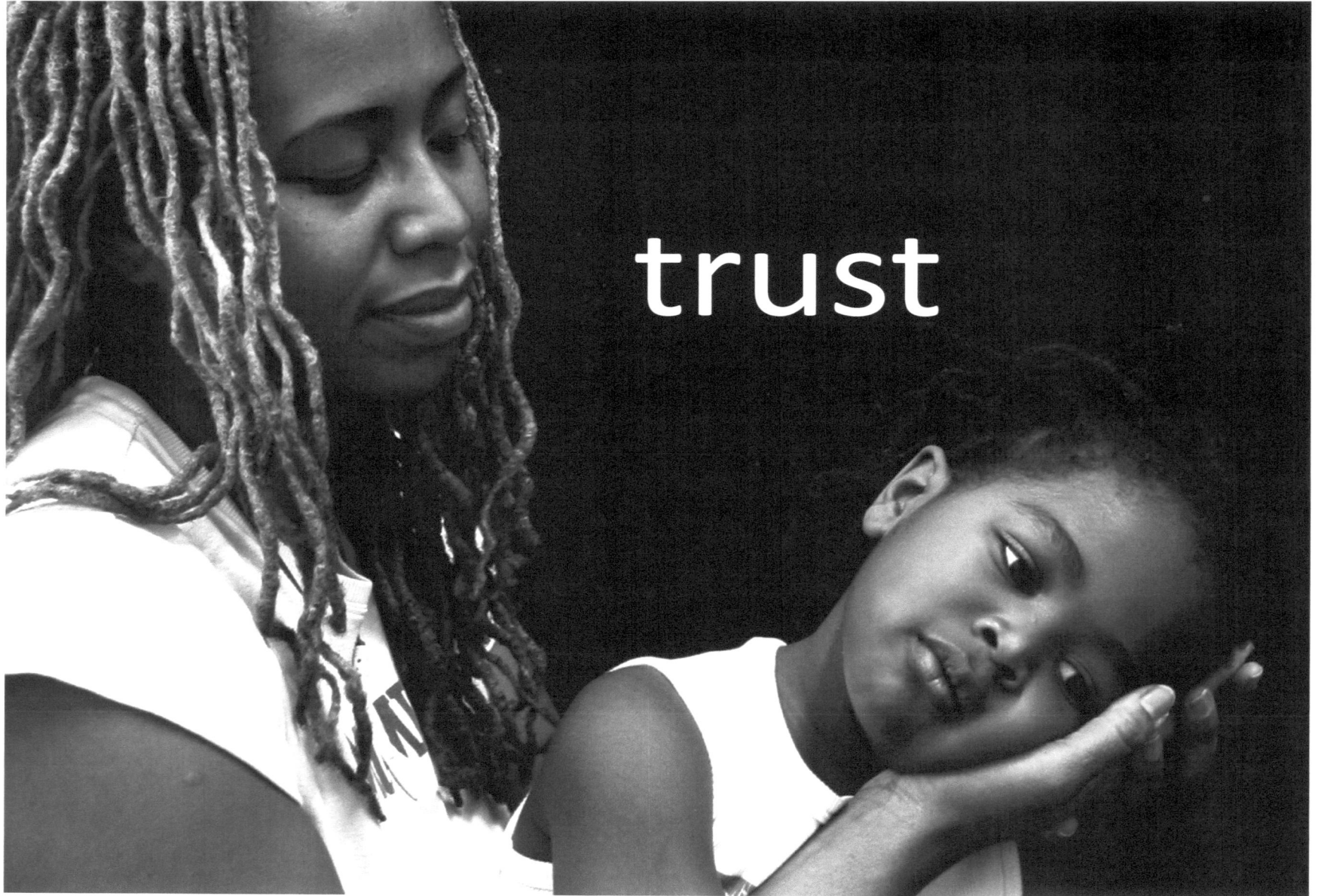

trust

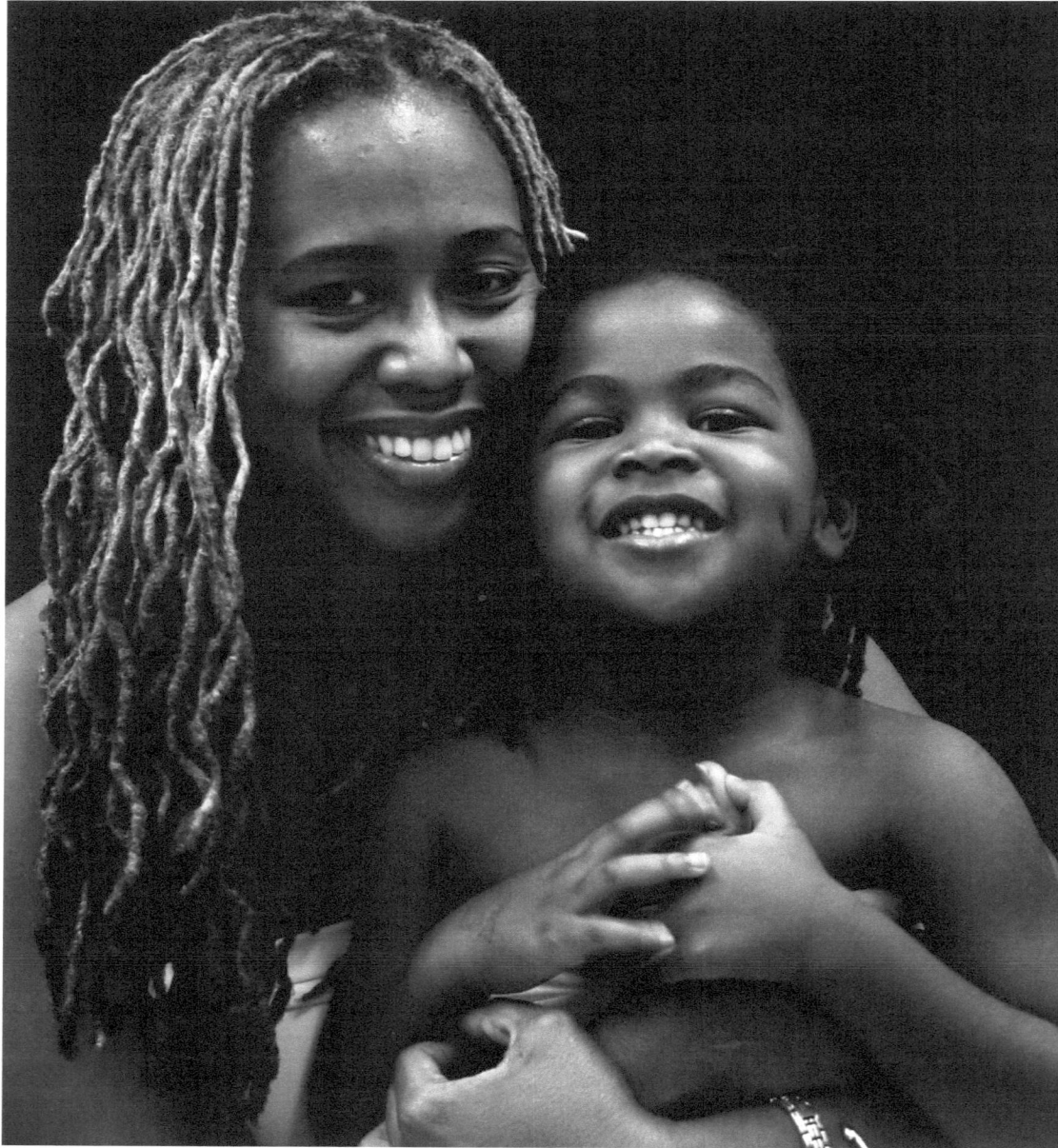

About the Photos

The state fire inspector told me there were too many photos on the walls of my thriving birth center as he carried out our annual inspection in 2006. Too many photos! I was incensed. Did he not understand the meaning and significance of every one of those snapshots and images? These were *my* babies, *my* mommies and *my* families and they had adorned the walls for years. We were renowned for our tapestry of wall-to-wall pictures and as we prepared to open a second clinic I struggled to come up with a way to continue the legacy of proudly displaying the literal 'fruits of our labor" in the new building. Then Alejandra Sarmiento walked into my life. A young mother herself, she had experienced a birth center birth, was midwife-friendly and had an amazing talent as a photographer. I immediately knew that she could solve my problem. We engaged some of our current patients in the idea of a photo shoot to create framed art for our new clinic. The response was overwhelming. Women, husbands, babies duly presented themselves, some nervous, tentative, embarrassed, and coy; some outrageous, dynamic, exuberant and wild. By the end of the sessions though, everyone was transformed, touched and inspired and I realized that I had uncovered something so precious that the only word I could find to describe it was - beautiful!

What is it about these women that are portrayed here? Why did I specifically choose their photos over others? It was difficult to decide but ultimately each person represents a triumph over the possibility of statistics to be truth, of data to define who we are. I wanted pregnant women to be able to see themselves fully represented for once; beautiful in all sizes, shapes, hues, blemishes and marks (not one of these images has been altered). I wanted everyone to be able to absorb the profound magnificence of pregnancy, birth and babies and be inspired to reclaim health for themselves and for their loved ones as well as to support healthy pregnancy for all.

This book developed as a way to tell the stories of the African American women in my practice who, just like the Caucasian, Asian and Hispanic women that I serve, carry their babies healthily to term. The application of The JJ Way® maternal child health system in a universal fashion has produced, against the odds, consistently positive outcomes for women of color in this clinic. These words and photos have captured that work and portray a cross-section of women and families who have experienced this method and achieved perfection in pregnancy, The JJ Way®.

Confidence (page 9). Statistics point to the fact that women who weigh less than 110 lbs before pregnancy are at risk for pre-term labor and birth. Underweight women may be malnourished and not able to support a growing fetus. Also small-breasted women often have a sense that they will be unable to successfully breastfeed their baby. Finally, the collective fear in America that the baby won't "fit", especially in smaller women undermines everyone's sense of trust in the reliability of nature to take its course. This second-time mom exudes the confidence of a woman who knows she can trust herself and her body to do this awesome job. She carried this pregnancy to term, just like her first one, produced almost 8 lb babies each time and successfully breastfed both girls. A busy executive with a large non-profit agency, she negated the fact that

even college-educated Black women are represented disproportionately in the statistics for poor birth outcomes.

Pride (page 12). Due to increased chances of diabetes and high blood pressure, pre-pregnant weight is a factor in poor perinatal health. I am convinced that self-esteem is another. The JJ Way® recognizes the importance of boosting and supporting a healthy self-image and incorporates time with each patient to ensure this is done. This woman in her seventh month, with her third child, glows with pride, comfortable and confident that in this case, size does not matter. She went on to deliver a healthy, full-term 7 lb baby without any problems.

Peace (page 15). Waiting on number four, the probability of another early baby was high. This young mom (23 years old) had three previous pre-term deliveries. She had seen an obstetrician for the other pregnancies but attended our clinic for prenatal care with this baby. Understanding from all of our staff that another early baby was not an option, she duly carried her baby to term and delivered the biggest baby she had ever had. Her photos portray the absolute serenity of knowing, even at seven months, that she and her baby were safe this time.

Power (page 17) was expecting her first baby. A smart young woman, she had an air of good common sense and was well supported by her family. Her images portray the way she carried her baby – with absolutely no room for anything but the finest outcome for herself and her baby. And so it was.

Triumph (page 21). Totally set up to expect another poor outcome, this mother had experienced severe pre-eclampsia (high blood pressure in pregnancy) resulting in an emergency Cesarean section of a very premature infant at 28 weeks in her last pregnancy. She was convinced she would have problems with all subsequent pregnancies. Her willingness to listen and follow my advice, coupled with collaborative care using The JJ Way® and our back-up OB physician bought her safely and beautifully to term. The photos speak for themselves.

Majestic (page 30) presented to my clinic initially, desperate and 'strung-out' on crack cocaine. She knew she needed help, she wanted a healthy baby but she couldn't battle the addiction on her own. After being assessed by our local High-Risk Perinatal Clinic, being admitted as an inpatient at a rehabilitation center, and becoming clean again we were able to welcome her back to our care. She subsequently carried her baby girl all the way to 39 weeks of pregnancy, delivered naturally and has become the mother she always dreamed of being. A hard life of insurmountable pain, yet new hope was generated by the transformational power of pregnancy and birth.

Delight (page 33). What joy to see an expectant mother so excited about the prospect of her soon-to-be-born baby. There is peace and confidence exuding from her; she knows that all is well and that once again she can finish the job in hand.

Anticipation (page 35). A first time momma whose photos reveal that occasional apprehension that is present for all of us. Never having experienced a pregnancy and birth before leaves one without a frame of reference. The JJ Way® has purposely incorporated the time needed for women to be able to ask all their questions, assuage their fears and gain confidence and understanding of what to expect. As the third trimester looms, typically women and families begin to feel the pressure of the upcoming birth and what it will mean for everyone involved. This woman grew in such confidence, made it to term and delivered naturally in the hospital despite developing high blood pressure at

38 weeks. Her strength and resolve carried her through to the triumph of a healthy outcome for herself and her baby.

Faith (page 39) is clearly apparent in this photo. A previous Cesarean section left this mom determined to have a vaginal delivery with this upcoming baby. She knew exactly what to do and availed herself of all the information and support necessary to achieve her goal. Her photos demonstrate the peace of believing and trusting in the power of your body to do what it inherently knows how to do.

Possibility (page 45) shines forth from this woman who was a bundle of nerves in the beginning of her pregnancy but settled into the groove of motherhood long before her baby was born. She came to our practice late in pregnancy after having been 'discharged' from an Obstetrician's office due to insurance issues. Providing prenatal care to any woman who has a need is an integral part of The JJ Way® and why we see such amazing outcomes.

Bonding (page 51) is a key component of The JJ Way® system. It is imperative that the pregnant woman herself bonds prenatally to the baby, but it is equally important that immediate family and friends do so too. When all concerned take on the 'team' effort of working towards a healthy outcome then invariably that's what happens.

Satisfaction (page 65). The supreme look of contentment, gratification and pleasure exude from this new mother. An easy pregnancy, a four hour natural delivery and effortless breastfeeding have blessed this first time momma.

Devotion (page 68). A teen mom, age seventeen, totally committed to the very best for her baby, just like her own mother (page 70) who was also a teen mom at age fourteen. Throughout the pregnancy, birth and breastfeeding this family has rallied around their new addition and provided every possible means of support. Every baby should be this loved.

Tenderness (page 71). Love envelopes this mother and baby as displayed in these caring moments that eventually bring forth a tentative smile. Unknown to any of us, this mom was newly pregnant again at the time of the photo shoot.

Hope (page 73) for the future. One of our juicy babies!

Commitment (page 74). Another momma freed from the vice grip of drug addiction. Cleaned up in early pregnancy, she completed a residential rehabilitation and continued her prenatal care at the center. After an arduous 24 hours in labor she was delivered by Cesarean section of a beautiful healthy boy. Courage and determination continue to drive her to be the best mother she can be for her baby.

Joy (page 78). Mother to an eleven year old, this unexpected pregnancy was an added pressure in this woman's already stressful life. She came to my center simply to receive the basic care but quickly determined that she was going to embrace the opportunity of birthing naturally, and threw herself wholeheartedly into our program. She ultimately had one of the most moving and inspiring births that I have ever had the honor of attending. As I watched her work through her contractions, supported and encouraged by her two brothers (who actually thought their only purpose

was to provide the transportation to the center that early morning and had *no* idea of the significance of their being present), I witnessed and experienced a phenomenal shift, a development, a transition, the absolute bonding of a family right in front of my eyes. It was a pivotal moment for us all.

Spirit (page 81) describes this young mother of two rambunctious boys. Despite all of the intricacies of her very hectic life she has made a stand for her twins and handles everything that comes at her with verve, energy and determination. Although she was not a patient of mine during her pregnancy she became an employee when her babies were six months old. Today she supports the women in the practice as she works as a medical assistant and as an encouragement and role model to other single moms.

Connection (page 82). Father and son.

Innocence and Promise (pages 84 and 85). Our children, our future.

Trust (page 86). A beautiful home-birthed baby, bonded, nurtured, loved. This woman chose to deliver her baby using a midwife because she wanted the opportunity to experience her birth, her way. The ease with which this little (9lb) baby came into the world was testimony to her parents making the right choice, for all of them. As a midwife I know the power in that decision. Three years later these photos show the legacy of that optimal beginning. This mother and daughter represent the promise of a brighter future for our collective health. Let us once again trust our bodies, our mothers, our sisters, our daughters and ultimately ourselves. Our babies are dying – it is time for us to stand up and say **_enough!_**

_____

Commonsense Childbirth Inc.

In 1998 I received the confirmation letter from the Internal Revenue Service that I had been awarded status as a federal non-profit Corporation under section 501(c)3 and Commonsense Childbirth Inc was born. Since then, we have served thousands of women who would have faltered or fallen down along the road to securing quality health care. Our vision then was that every person had the opportunity to have a healthy baby, and that no one was turned away.

Our mission remains to inspire change in maternal child health care systems; to re-empower the birthing mother, father, family and community by supporting the providers, practitioners and agencies that are charged with their care.

We aim to improve birth outcomes and save lives by offering training and certification programs for healthcare professionals, para-professionals, maternity care systems and medical institutions interested in creating perinatal safety for at-risk populations. We focus on safety, quality and workforce development in support of our vision for equitable maternity care.

We use The JJ Way® and the midwifery model of care, to achieve our health equity goals. Low birth weight prematurity, poor maternal and infant health and deaths are particularly high among Black people regardless of socioeconomic status, insurance status, education or citizenship.

We use The JJ Way® to grow and support the perinatal workforce to serve and support the communities that they deeply care about. Our training programs reach health professionals across the spectrum - doctors, midwives, nurses, health educators, childbirth educators, lactation educators, social workers, community health workers - and the general public. Our reach includes health and educational institutions, public health and community-based organizations and collectives.

Now our evidence-based clinics, programs, training and accreditation are scaling nationally and although the photos in this book were taken in 2007, they represent what we have stood for from the onset. Since our first study in 2006 our research and statistics continue to prove that we have all but eradicated prematurity and low birth weight babies while maintaining health and increasing breastfeeding rates among the birthing people that we serve. Our growing body of trained and certified midwives and perinatal professionals deliver consistent and reliable results with fidelity to The JJ Way® model and significantly impact their communities and their own development as we together focus on growing and operationalizing the community birth infrastructure that is essential to all of our futures.

As a non-profit organization we depend on donations, grants, and in-kind support. A percentage of the proceeds from the sale of this book will go towards continuing the work of our clinics, our midwifery and educational programs, our policy work and the sharing and scaling of The JJ Way® Maternal Child Health System throughout the United States. Your support is appreciated and please go to www.commonsensechildbirth.org if you would like to donate.

Endorsements

"Beautiful!", gives America an intimate view of the diversity and uniqueness in pregnancy. Within the pages of *Beautiful!* we see possibilities, so important when the sacredness of pregnancy is still misunderstood. This book needs to be on every shelf in America, to empower women to glow with a healthy pregnancy.

Shafia M. Monroe,
Midwife, founder International Center for Traditional Childbearing www.blackmidwives.org

---

Encouragement. That is what you will find within the pages of this book. You will begin to believe again in healthy non-surgically orchestrated births of joyous little human beings. You will begin to understand that pregnancy complications and infant mortality can be addressed directly and without pretense. You will begin to dream about a world where every woman can deliver a healthy, happy child regardless of social constraints, economic scarcity or ethnicity.

Jennie Joseph prods us along with wondrous images and hard evidence. She encourages us to believe. She encourages us to pay attention and understand that we do, in fact hold the key to reducing the disparities that currently define pregnancy, childbirth and the neonatal period. She urges us to wake up and ask for, to stand up and expect, that our babies be born healthy and at term in a natural way. Every difficult journey has a long path, but Jennie Joseph offers a light along that path to illuminate the way back to understanding pregnancy and childbirth as a wholesome, natural phenomenon, not a medical illness. The JJ Way® offers all of this and more. Read for yourself and be… encouraged.

Deanna Wathington, MD, MPH
Director, Public Health Practice Program College of Public Health University of South Florida

At 19 years old, all I knew was that I was pregnant and I wanted a healthy pregnancy and a healthy baby. I sought someone to care for me on a level that is virtually unheard of in the United States. I sought someone who would treat me as a person separate from the baby that I was carrying, but also to hold my baby's health to be as important as I did. I sought someone to care for me and my unborn child without prejudice. I sought someone to guide me into making my own decisions surrounding my pregnancy and birth experience. I sought a provider to treat me as a young woman who was pregnant, not a patient who was ill. I found Jennie Joseph. I found exactly what I was looking for. Jennie has touched and inspired my life, the life of my child, and the lives of so many others who, after having experienced The JJ Way®, would have it no other way. The JJ Way® is an inspiration to the practice of not only midwifery, but to the medical profession as a whole. It inspires the patient to believe that they have the ability to invest in their own health and have excellent outcomes.

Five years after walking into Jennie Joseph's 'The Birth Place' practice, I am now an RN and can see the effects of using the The JJ Way® to relate to patients, even in a non-obstetrical setting. It takes a unique concept such as the The JJ Way® to encourage people to take charge of their health and consequently, their lives.

Temperance Taylor, RN
Mother to 5 year old Kaleb

Life's rhythm is a perfect balance of beginnings and endings. Pregnancy signals a time for two lives to become one breath. Every healthy baby enriches their family, community, and beyond. Birthing a child is hands-down one of the most miraculous human experiences. Ensuring the well-being of a child is a privilege and honor that I have been blessed to have as a Mother, Pediatrician, wellness expert, and philanthropist. Jennie captures the essences of victory in each image of Mothers who re-birthed themselves throughout the birthing experience. Join me in celebrating life The JJ Way® and greet your unexpected challenges in royal style.

Toni Moody, MD
Pediatrician, Founder of Health Masters Club, a non-profit charity dedicated to ensuring our children's well-being and the Collaborative for Healthy Breasts 2020.

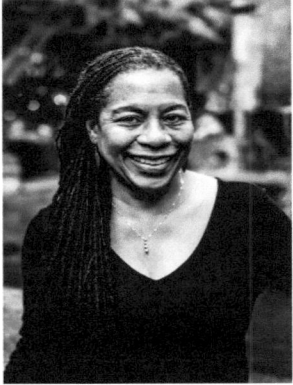

Jennie Joseph is a well-respected health advocate for women and newborn babies. A British-trained midwife, Jennie has become one of the world's most respected midwives and authorities on maternal health: healthy pregnancies, healthy deliveries, healthy postpartum and healthy babies. She's become a true advocate for systematic reform that puts women, babies and families first in healthcare; before profit, convenience and the numerous societal reasons America trails other developed nations in safe maternity care. Jennie's common-sense approach and consistently better outcomes have won her the attention of global news media and brought her invitations to speak all over the world.

She has worked extensively in European hospitals, American birth centers, clinics, and homebirth environments. She has been instrumental in the regulation of Florida midwives since the 1990s and has been involved in midwifery education in the US since 1995. She is the former chair of Florida's State Council of Licensed Midwives. Currently, she is the founder of the United States first nationally-accredited, private midwifery school owned by a Black woman - Commonsense Childbirth School of Midwifery. Alongside The Birth Place, her world renowned birth center, maternity care center and Easy Access Clinic™ in Central Florida, she also heads up the National Perinatal Task Force which is a national branch of Commonsense Childbirth designed to support and develop the perinatal workforce through collective care and collective leadership.

Jennie never set out for accolades or influence. In fact, she remains driven today by the one thing that brought her to maternal health care: she loves helping families and growing the maternity care workforce. This care for others amid mounting frustrations from witnessing unnecessary traumas and unethical care resulting in harm and death caused her to speak out and advocate for a better way. Calling out the historical and systemic racism, classism and gender discrimination that permeates the field, Jennie has provided immediate, practical, and evidence-based solutions that have contributed to her continued success in serving women safely and helping others across the globe do the same.

Jennie has pressed for linkages and collaboration with other public and private agencies in an effort to maintain continuity of care for the safety of her clients but also in order to bridge the gap between America's maternity care practitioners. She has developed and administers perinatal professional training and certification programs to address the health care provider shortage, diversify the maternal child health (MCH) workforce and address persistent racial and class disparities in birth outcomes. There are both quantitative and qualitative studies underway regarding Jennie's work as well as continuous reviews of the impact of her clinical and educational programs. Jennie's model of health care, The JJ Way®, provides an evidence-based system to deliver MCH services which improve health, reduce costs and produce better outcomes all round.

Jennie's efforts have allowed her to speak to doctors and other practitioners, policy makers, including members of the U.S. Congress in which she has testified at Congressional briefings on Capitol Hill, as well as serving as a regular presenter at maternal-child health conferences and organizations around the world. She has given a multitude of media interviews on these important topics and serves in leadership positions amongst U.S. and international midwives movements and organizations. She was honored to be named as one of twelve women for TIME magazine Woman of the Year 2022.

Jennie firmly believes in safe, quality, equitable care for every person, every time and works tirelessly to support the systems, providers and agencies charged with delivering that type of care. She considers that she is helping to operationalize the community birth and perinatal infrastructure by returning trusted providers to the heart of their communities. In the meantime this quote by Jennie sums it up - "Until women and their loved ones feel that they have enough knowledge and agency to be part of the decisions around their care, and until they have access to the education and support that they are lacking, they will continue to be at risk."